D1203087

The Radiology of
Orthopaedic Implants

MCP HAHNEMANN UNIVERSITY
HAHNEMANN LIBRARY

The Radiology of Orthopaedic Implants

AN ATLAS OF TECHNIQUES AND ASSESSMENT

—

Andrew A. Freiberg, M.D.

Assistant Professor
Chief, Adult Reconstruction Service
Section of Orthopaedic Surgery
The University of Michigan Medical School
Ann Arbor, Michigan

Foreword by William Martel, M.D.

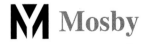 Mosby

A Harcourt Health Sciences Company

St. Louis   London   Philadelphia   Sydney   Toronto

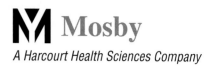

Mosby

A Harcourt Health Sciences Company

Editor-in-Chief: Richard Lampert
Production Manager: Frank Polizzano
Illustration Specialist: Peg Shaw
Indexer: Dennis Dolan

Copyright © 2001 by Mosby, Inc.

All rights reserved. No part of this publication may be reproduced or transmitted in any form or by any means, electronic or mechanical, including photocopy, recording, or any information storage and retrieval system, without permission in writing from the publisher.

Permission to photocopy or reproduce solely for internal or personal use is permitted for libraries or other users registered with the Copyright Clearance Center, provided that the base fee of $4.00 per chapter plus $.10 per page is paid directly to the Copyright Clearance Center, 222 Rosewood Drive, Danvers, Massachusetts 01923. This consent does not extend to other kinds of copying, such as copying for general distribution, for advertising or promotional purposes, for creating new collected works, or for resale.

Mosby, Inc.
A Harcourt Health Sciences Company
11830 Westline Industrial Drive
St. Louis, Missouri 63146

Printed in the United States of America.

Library of Congress Cataloging-in-Publication Data

The radiology of orthopaedic implants: an atlas of techniques and assessment / [edited by] Andrew A. Freiberg; foreword by William Martel.

p.   cm.

ISBN 0–323–00222–6

1. Orthopedic implants—Radiography—Atlases.   2. Radiography in orthopedics—Atlases.   3. Musculoskeletal system—Diseases—Diagnosis—Atlases.   4. Joints—Radiography—Atlases. I. Freiberg, Andrew A.

[DNLM: 1. Arthrography—methods—Atlases.   2. Joint Prosthesis—Atlases. 3. Bone and Bones—radiography—Atlases.   4. Orthopedic Fixation Devices—Atlases. WE 17 R1295 2001]

RD755.5.R33 2001
617.4′70592—dc21   2001018323

01 02 03 04 05 9 8 7 6 5 4 3 2 1

To my loving wife, Dee, our wonderful children, Stephen and Benjamin, and my father and late mother whose love and support have been immeasurable

Contributors

——

Ronald S. Adler, Ph.D., M.D.
Professor, Cornell University Joan and Sanford I. Weill Medical College and Graduate School of Medical Sciences; Attending Radiologist, Hospital for Special Surgery, New York, New York
Ultrasound of Joint Replacements

Daniel J. Berry, M.D.
Associate Professor of Orthopaedic Surgery, Mayo Medical School; Consultant, Orthopaedic Surgery, Mayo Clinic, Rochester, Minnesota
Hydroxyapatite-Coated Femoral Components

James E. Carpenter, M.D.
Associate Professor, The University of Michigan Shoulder Group, Section of Orthopaedic Surgery, The University of Michigan Medical School, Ann Arbor, Michigan
The Shoulder

Shirley Chow, M.D.
Fellow-Associate, Department of Radiology, The University of Iowa Hospitals and Clinics, Iowa City, Iowa
Foot and Ankle Implants

Peter A. Devane, M.B.Ch.B., F.R.A.C.S., M.Sc.
Senior Lecturer in Orthopaedic Surgery, Wellington School of Medicine; Consultant, Orthopaedic Surgery, Wellington Hospital, Wellington, New Zealand
Measurement of Polyethylene Wear in Total Hip Joint Replacement

Georges Y. El-Khoury, M.D., S.A.C.R.
Professor of Radiology and Orthopaedics, The University of Iowa College of Medicine; Vice-Chairman, Department of Radiology, The University of Iowa Hospitals and Clinics, Iowa City, Iowa
Foot and Ankle Implants

Andrew A. Freiberg, M.D.
Assistant Professor and Chief, Adult Reconstruction Service, Section of Orthopaedic Surgery, The University of Michigan Medical School, Ann Arbor, Michigan
Radiology of Total Hip Replacement

Gregory J. Golladay, M.D.
Assistant in Orthopaedic Surgery, Massachusetts General Hospital, Boston, Massachusetts
Radiology of Total Hip Replacement

Gregory P. Graziano, M.D.
Associate Professor, Section of Orthopaedic Surgery and Neurosurgery, University of Michigan Medical School, Ann Arbor, Michigan
Spinal Instrumentation

David J. Hak, M.D.
Assistant Professor, Department of Orthopaedic Surgery, University of California, Davis, Medical Center, Sacramento, California
Trauma

Brian R. Hallstrom, M.D.
Assistant in Orthopaedic Surgery, Massachusetts General Hospital, Boston, Massachusetts
Radiology of Total Hip Replacement

J. Geoffrey Horne, M.B.Ch.B., F.R.C.S.(C), F.R.A.C.S.
Professor of Surgery, Wellington School of Medicine, Wellington, New Zealand
Measurement of Polyethylene Wear in Total Hip Joint Replacement

Peter J. L. Jebson, M.D.
Assistant Professor, Section of Orthopaedic Surgery, Division of Elbow, Hand Microsurgery, University of Michigan Medical School, Ann Arbor, Michigan
Orthopaedic Implants of the Elbow, Wrist, and Hand

John E. Kuhn, M.D.
Assistant Professor, The University of Michigan Shoulder Group, Section of Orthopaedic Surgery, The University of Michigan Medical School, Ann Arbor, Michigan
The Shoulder

David S. Kwon, M.D.
Clinical Instructor of Radiology, Tufts University School of Medicine, Boston; Orthopaedic Radiologist, Hallmark Imaging Associates, P.C., Melrose-Wakefield Hospital, Melrose, Massachusetts
Musculoskeletal Imaging and Interventions

Seth S. Leopold, M.D.
Fellow in Adult Reconstructive Orthopaedics, Rush Medical College of Rush University, Chicago, Illinois
Impaction Allografting with Cement for Femoral Component Revision

Dean S. Louis, M.D.
Professor of Surgery and Chief of Orthopaedic Hand Surgery, Section of Orthopaedic Surgery, University of Michigan Medical Center, Ann Arbor, Michigan
Orthopaedic Implants of the Elbow, Wrist, and Hand

David C. Markel, M.D.
Assistant Clinical Professor, Orthopaedic Surgery, Wayne State University School of Medicine, Detroit; Chief, Orthopaedic Surgery, Providence Hospital, Southfield, Michigan
Primary and Revision Arthroplasty of the Knee

Brian J. McGrory, M.D.
Clinical Associate Professor, Department of Orthopaedic Surgery and Rehabilitation, University of Vermont School of Medicine, Burlington, Vermont
Hydroxyapatite-Coated Femoral Components

Arthur H. Newberg, M.D.
Professor of Radiology and Orthopaedics, Tufts University School of Medicine;
Chief, Musculoskeletal Imaging, Department of Radiology, New England Baptist
Hospital, Boston, Massachusetts
Musculoskeletal Imaging and Interventions

Joel S. Newman, M.D.
Assistant Professor of Radiology, Tufts University School of Medicine; Associate
Director, Musculoskeletal Imaging, Department of Radiology, New England
Baptist Hospital, Boston, Massachusetts
Musculoskeletal Imaging and Interventions

Aaron G. Rosenberg, M.D.
Professor of Orthopaedic Surgery, Rush Medical College of Rush University,
Chicago, Illinois
Impaction Allografting with Cement for Femoral Component Revision

Charles L. Saltzman, M.D.
Associate Professor, Department of Orthopaedic Surgery and Associate Professor,
Department of Biomedical Engineering, The University of Iowa, College of
Medicine, Iowa City, Iowa
Foot and Ankle Implants

Ethan J. Schock, M.D.
Resident, University of Michigan Medical School; Ann Arbor, Michigan
Spinal Instrumentation

Jon K. Sekiya, M.D.
Chief Resident, Section of Orthopaedic Surgery, University of Michigan Medical
Center, Ann Arbor, Michigan
Sports Medicine: Implants of Knee Ligament Repair and Reconstructive Surgery

Adam W. J. Tonakie, M.D.
South Coast Radiology, Queensland, Australia
Nuclear Medicine Imaging

Richard Wahl, M.D.
Director, Division of Nuclear Medicine; Vice Chairman for Technology and
Development, Department of Radiology, Johns Hopkins Medical Institutions,
Baltimore, Maryland
Nuclear Medicine Imaging

Edward M. Wojtys, M.D.
Professor, Section of Orthopaedic Surgery, University of Michigan Medical School,
Ann Arbor, Michigan
Sports Medicine: Implants of Knee Ligament Repair and Reconstructive Surgery

Foreword

—

Many thousands of orthopaedic reconstructive and internal fixation procedures are performed annually. A variety of related surgical techniques and hardware/implant devices have also evolved. In addition, new medical imaging and interventional techniques have been developed for preoperative and postoperative evaluation.

This excellent book, *The Radiology of Orthopaedic Implants*, describes in detail the often complex related orthopaedic procedures. It focuses on preoperative and postoperative appearances and complications. Written largely in the form of an atlas, it comprises 14 chapters. Each skeletal region is treated separately by nationally recognized experts who are extremely knowledgeable and have extensive experience with these surgical techniques. There are also invaluable chapters dealing with trauma, sports medicine, femoral impaction allografting with cement, measurement of polyethylene wear in total hip replacement, and hydroxyapatite-coated femoral components. Excellent chapters are included that deal with musculoskeletal imaging, such as computed tomography and magnetic resonance imaging, and with interventional techniques, ultrasonography, and nuclear scintigraphy. The radiographs and illustrations are excellent. The accompanying legends clearly describe the significant features and how to recognize specific complications. The text in each chapter is brief and informative.

Dr. Freiberg has given us a superb and comprehensive book on a very important subject. It is on the cutting edge of our knowledge and in many instances fills a void in our current medical literature. This surely will become a classic reference, which will be invaluable for all physicians treating these patients, particularly orthopaedic surgeons and radiologists.

WILLIAM MARTEL, M.D.
Fred Jenner Hodges Professor of Radiology Emeritus
University of Michigan Medical School
Ann Arbor, Michigan

Preface

—

Orthopaedic surgeons and radiologists work within the same institutions, but often in parallel. There is a distinct language to the accurate description of orthopaedic implants. The major focus of *The Radiology of Orthopaedic Implants* is to bring our two specialties together to improve patient care.

The description of the variety of orthopaedic procedures combined with the huge array of available implants seems daunting. We understand the clinical and radiographic natural history of many orthopaedic diseases. The accurate interpretation of abnormal findings and implant failures is also an extremely important aspect of patient care. Radiologists and orthopaedic surgeons must also come together with a common language to describe musculoskeletal conditions.

One unique aspect of orthopaedic radiology is the use of implants. Implant applications can vary along with a wide variety of types. There are many implants, and there are many ways for them to fail. Early recognition and accurate communication about these abnormalities are critical. Radiographic changes can precede clinical symptoms, and radiographic surveillance can thereby prevent morbidity.

This atlas is organized into both specialty and procedural sections. There are contributions from recognized experts in the field—all of whom share their experience and knowledge.

I hope this text provides a foundation for better collaboration between orthopaedic surgeons and radiologists and ultimately improves the care we provide.

Acknowledgments

—

I would like to recognize the unselfish contributions of my many orthopaedic and radiology colleagues. Their dedication to this project has been outstanding.

Special acknowledgment should also go to Karen Edwards and Michelle Davis whose commitments to organization and completion are truly appreciated.

Contents

——

1

Musculoskeletal Imaging and Interventions

DAVID S. KWON

JOEL S. NEWMAN

ARTHUR H. NEWBERG

Radiography, fluoroscopy, cross-sectional imaging, nuclear scintigraphy, and minimally invasive procedures such as joint aspiration and arthrography are tools available for the evaluation of orthopaedic implants. Diagnostic and therapeutic imaging strategies and techniques available to the pre- and postoperative orthopaedic patient are addressed. There is specific focus on the techniques, positioning, and standardization of plain radiographs, the technique and interpretation of joint arthrography and aspiration, and the potential roles of computed tomography and magnetic resonance imaging. Complications as well as normal variants that may be mistaken for complications are demonstrated in pictorial format.

Radiography

Several hundred thousand arthroplasties are performed worldwide each year, including an estimated 120,000 total hip arthroplasties and more than 100,000 total knee replacements that are performed in the United States alone.[1-3] An adjunct to the clinical examination, conventional and digitally acquired images of orthopaedic implants can provide a relatively inexpensive and generally reliable means of assessing postoperative interaction between prosthetic components and native bone (Table 1-1). Potential complications that may occur after surgery can be identified, particularly loosening, infection, component wear, component migration, and similar abnormalities. Routine protocols that are performed before surgery of the hip, shoulder, and knee are addressed, as are protocols related to the use of postoperative films.

PREOPERATIVE HIP RADIOGRAPHS

Routine preoperative views should include an anteroposterior (AP) view of the pelvis, centered at a point halfway between the hips, an AP view of the affected hip, including the proximal two thirds of the femur, and a modified Lauenstein lateral view (Fig. 1-1), which is performed by placing the patient in an oblique, nearly lateral position on the affected side, with the hip and knee in flexion. The central ray from the x-ray source is positioned at a point halfway between the anterosuperior iliac spine and the pubic symphysis. Less foreshortening of the femur occurs when using this method than occurs when using a modified frog-leg view of the hip,

Table 1–1   *Significance of Radiologic Findings in Uncemented Hip Prosthetics*

Finding	Incidence	Clinical Significance
Sclerosis at tip	Frequent	None
Sclerosis of calcar	Frequent	None
Resorption of calcar	Mild degrees common	None
Lucency < 2 mm	One third of cases	Occasional pain or loosening
Lucency > 2 mm		High incidence of loosening Consider infection
Early cartilage space loss		Infection, especially if pain or loss of subchondral cortex occurs
Late cartilage space loss		Exacerbation or development of osteoarthritis or other arthritis
Acetabular sclerosis	Frequent, if mild	Mild: asymptomatic Severe: may be symptomatic.

Adapted from Freedman MT. Radiol Clin North Am 1975, 13:45.

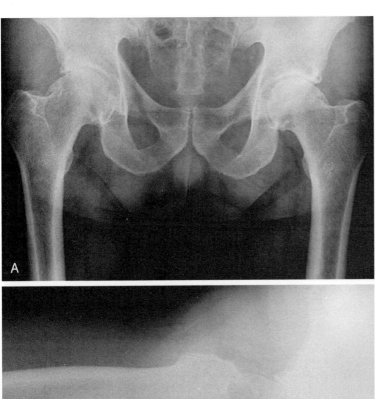

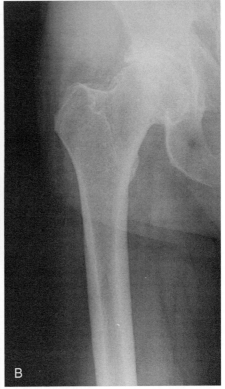

FIGURE 1–1 Routine preoperative hip radiographs in a 47-year-old patient with right hip pain. **A:** An AP view centered over the hips demonstrates osteoarthritis bilaterally. **B:** An AP view of the affected hip. **C:** A modified Lauenstein lateral x-ray. The hip joint and proximal femur should be demonstrated in the lateral position, with the greater trochanter superimposed on the femoral neck.

which is performed with the pelvis kept in an AP position and with the affected femur positioned obliquely at the hip.

POSTOPERATIVE HIP RADIOGRAPHS

Postoperative and follow-up films may include an AP view of the pelvis, centered between both hips, an AP view of the hip, including an AP view of the entire femoral stem, and a Lauenstein lateral view (Fig. 1–2). In the setting of stemless surface replacements and mold (cup) arthroplasties, some practitioners have suggested the inclusion of an AP view of the pelvis with the x-ray beam centered between the hips, an AP grid coordinate roentgenogram of the affected hip, a true lateral, and an oblique (Judet) view of the acetabulum.[4] The Judet view is performed with the patient in a 45-degree posterior oblique position either with the side of interest down (closest to the table), which demonstrates abnormalities of the posterior (ilioischial) column and anterior acetabular rim, or with the affected side up, which demonstrates the anterior (iliopubic) column and posterior acetabular rim (Fig. 1–3).[5] The importance of obtaining an image of the entire prosthetic stem cannot be overemphasized, as change in position, fracture of the component, motion, or infection can be readily overlooked (Fig. 1–4).

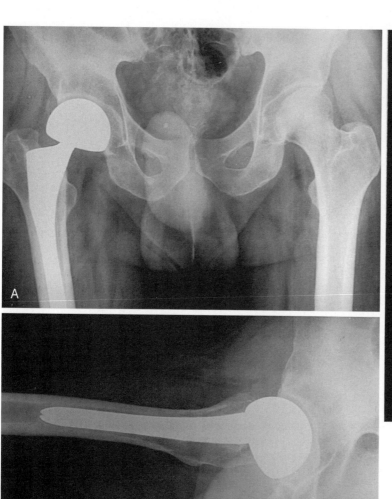

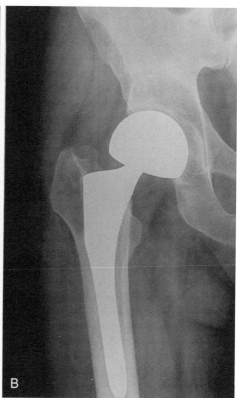

FIGURE 1–2 Routine radiographs taken after hip arthroplasty. **A:** The orthopaedic AP pelvis is centered between the hips to include as much of the femoral component as possible. **B:** An AP view of the affected hip with a bipolar prosthesis in place (note the inclusion of the entire femoral prosthetic stem). **C:** A modified Lauenstein lateral x-ray.

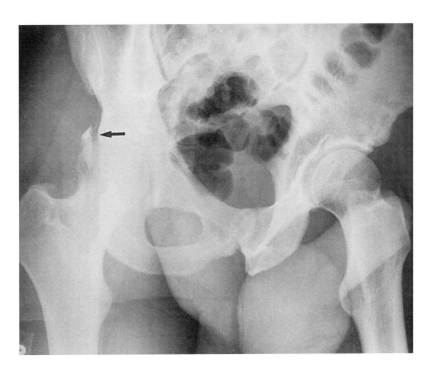

FIGURE 1–3 A Judet obturator oblique view of a native right hip demonstrates a posterior acetabular fracture (arrow) and no abnormality of the iliopubic bones.

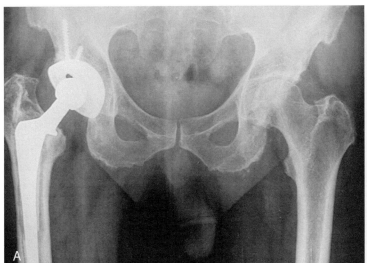
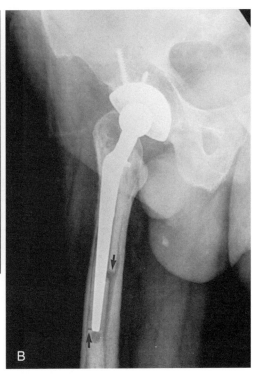

FIGURE 1–4 Fractured cement surrounding the femoral stem. **A:** The orthopaedic AP pelvis demonstrates a fracture of the cement along the medial aspect of the femoral stem. **B:** A modified Lauenstein x-ray includes the entire femoral stem and demonstrates cement fractures (arrows) adjacent to the femoral stem tip. The importance of obtaining an image of the entire stem is emphasized.

PREOPERATIVE KNEE RADIOGRAPHS

AP, lateral, intercondylar fossa (tunnel/notch) and patellar (skyline) views of the knee are routinely obtained preoperatively. Additionally, weightbearing AP views of the legs, including the hips and ankles, are obtained to assess the patient's mechanical axis. The mechanical axis is drawn from the center of the femoral head to the center of the ankle joint. An anatomic axis is determined by drawing lines through the long axis of the femoral and tibial shaft. The angle between the mechanical axis and the femoral axis is measured. During surgery, the femur is resected at the angle measured to provide the proper mechanical axis after placing intramedullary guides along the anatomic axis of the femur.

POSTOPERATIVE KNEE RADIOGRAPHS

AP, lateral, and patellar views should be obtained after knee surgery (Fig. 1–5). Allen and colleagues state that the mechanical axis should pass through the center or just medial to the center of the prosthetic knee and that the femoral component should be within 4 to 11 degrees of anatomic valgus.[11] On the lateral view, the femoral component should be parallel or nearly parallel to the long axis of the femur and should match the native contour of the femur. The tibial component should be horizontal or slightly downsloping posteriorly no more than 10 degrees. The alignment of the tibial prosthesis should be perpendicular to the shaft of the tibia on the AP projection. Ideally, the inferior edge of the patella should lie 10 to 30 mm from a line drawn parallel, extending from the tibial articulating surface.[12]

PREOPERATIVE SHOULDER RADIOGRAPHS

Views obtained of a preoperative shoulder may include AP views with the humeral head in internal as well as external rotation; an anterior oblique (scapular-Y) view, which is a true lateral view of the scapula and projects the humeral head so it is centered over the glenoid; and a posterior oblique (Grashey) view, which shows the glenohumeral joint in profile. The posterior oblique view is the true AP view of the shoulder, as it takes into account the 20 degrees or so of anterior tilt of the glenoid fossa that is not normally seen on standard AP projections. The axillary view may also supplement these images. Some practitioners believe that the anterior and posterior oblique views are all that are necessary for diagnosis of most shoulder abnormalities.

Preoperative plain film radiographs can assess bone stock, bone destruction, evidence of infection, osteophyte formation, and the relationship between the glenoid and the humeral head and can detect some abnormalities of the acromioclavicular joint. This is not to mention the potential of detecting soft-tissue and bone tumors and evidence of soft-tissue mineralization.[14] The internal and external rotation views may help in the detection of a Hill-Sachs lesion, the Grashey view in determining abnormalities of the glenohumeral articulation and expected cartilage space, and the anterior oblique view in assessing the acromial shape and the relationship between the glenoid and humerus in terms of subluxation or dislocation.

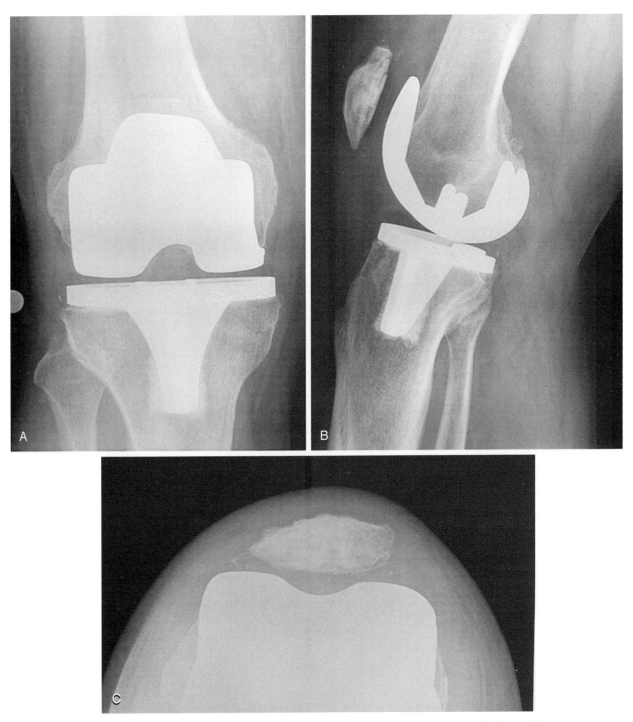

FIGURE 1–5　Routine radiographs after knee arthroplasty. **A:** An AP view of the knee. The tibial tray is perpendicular to the shaft of the tibia. **B:** A lateral view of the knee. The tibial tray is slightly downsloping posteriorly, but the angle of inclination generally should be less than 10 degrees. The patella should lie between 10 and 30 mm from its inferior edge to a line drawn parallel to the tibial surface. **C:** A patellar view of the knee.

POSTOPERATIVE SHOULDER RADIOGRAPHS

Routine follow-up and postoperative shoulder films parallel the preoperative radiographs. Anterior and posterior oblique as well as AP views of the humeral prosthesis may be obtained (Fig. 1–6).

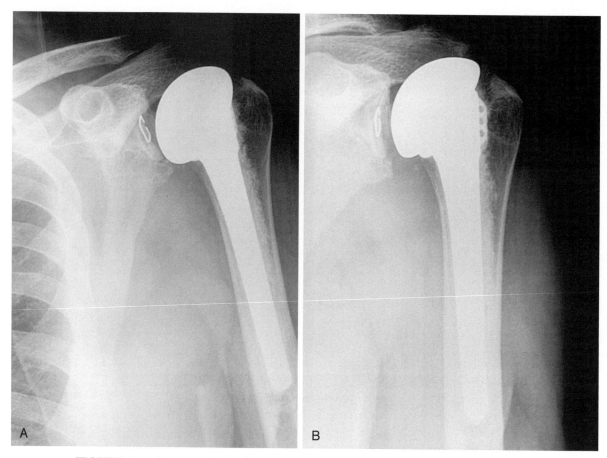

FIGURE 1–6   Routine radiographs after shoulder arthroplasty. **A:** An AP view of a left total shoulder arthroplasty. **B:** A posterior oblique (Grashey) view demonstrating the glenohumeral joint in profile.

Arthrography

Indications for joint aspiration and arthrography with respect to the postarthroplasty patient usually occur in the setting of possible infection or when there is persistent pain after joint replacement. Arthrographic features that suggest loosening or infection include the following:

1. Extension of contrast between the cement/bone or prosthetic/bone interface (Fig. 1–7)
2. Filling of para-articular cavities or sinus tracts (Fig. 1–8)
3. Lymphatic opacification (Fig. 1–9)

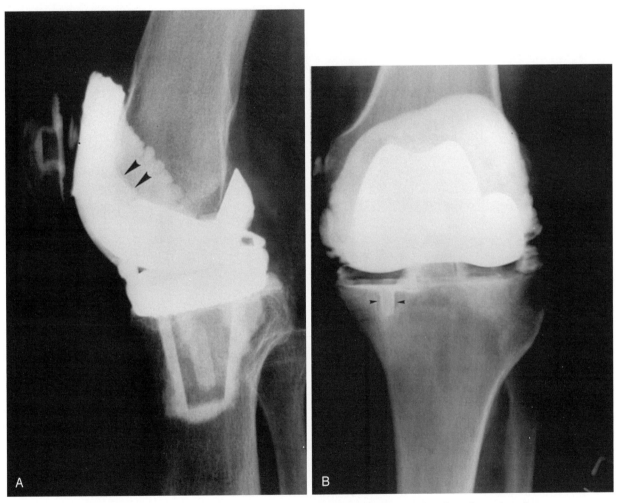

FIGURE 1–7 Extension of contrast between the bone/cement or prosthetic/bone interface during arthrography. Findings are suggestive of loosening and possible infection. **A:** Lateral knee radiograph during knee arthrography demonstrates a faint linear collection of contrast between the bone and the femoral prosthesis (arrowheads). **B:** An AP view of the knee of another patient during arthrography; contrast outlines the polyethylene medial components (arrowheads).

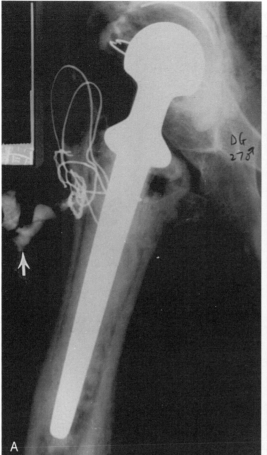

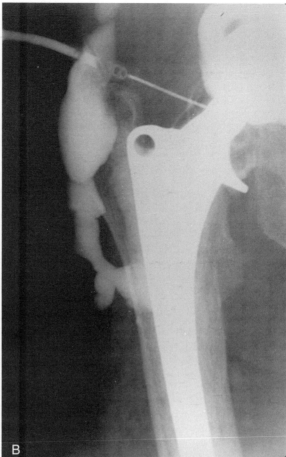

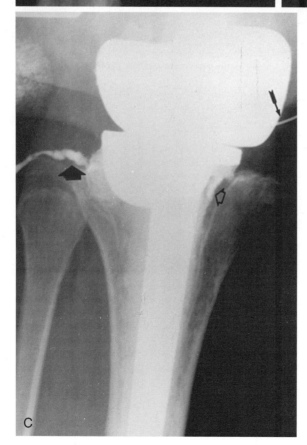

FIGURE 1–8 Contrast fills sinus tracts and cavities. **A:** An image obtained during arthrography of a right total hip arthroplasty in a 27-year-old male with hip pain. A sinus tract (white arrow) filled during arthrography in this patient in whom a culture of the joint revealed the presence of beta-hemolytic *Streptococcus*. **B:** Close-up of another patient who demonstrated a large periarticular sinus cavity that filled during arthrography of the hip. **C:** An AP view of a total knee arthroplasty demonstrates a sinus tract lateral to the tibia (widest arrow). The needle tip advances using a medial approach along the media facet, which is believed to be a shorter route to the joint than a lateral approach. The open arrow demonstrates contrast along the cement bone interface, also a sign of loosening and possible infection.

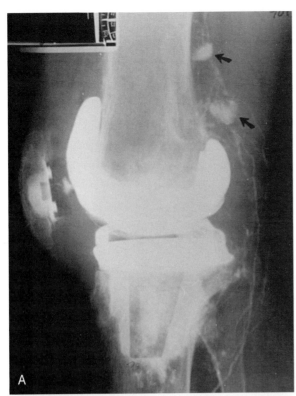

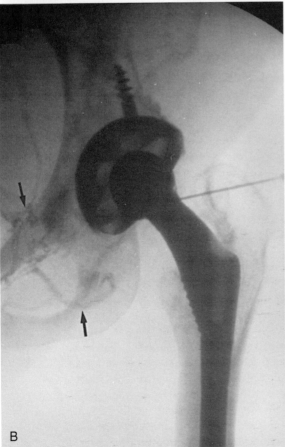

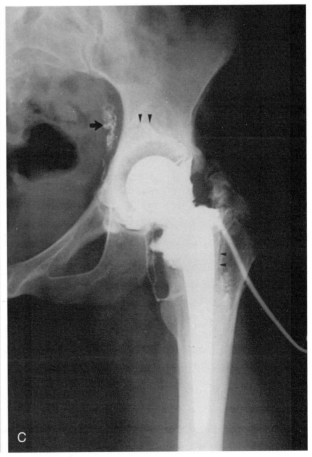

FIGURE 1–9 Examples of lymphatic opacification, which can be a normal variant found in some arthrograms due to limited joint capacity and distension of the joint with contrast or which can represent synovitis of the joint. It can also be a sign of infection, especially in the context of other arthrographic findings of loosening and infection. **A:** A lateral view of a total knee arthrogram with contrast outlining lymphatic vessels posteriorly (arrows) because of limited joint capacity. **B:** A negative image (the prosthesis is dark) of a left total hip arthrogram in a middle-aged female with hip pain. Arrows outline lymphatic vessels; limited joint capacity was present secondary to a large soft-tissue mass in the thigh, as seen on CT, which affected the hip joint. **C:** The filling of the lymphatic vessels (arrows) and areas of prosthetic loosening (arrowheads) in an infected total hip arthroplasty.

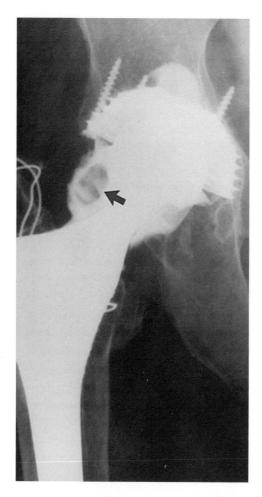

FIGURE 1–10 An intra-articular loose body (arrow) that was identified during routine hip arthrography.

Arthrography can also demonstrate intra-articular filling defects that may represent loose bodies, a potential cause of mechanical dysfunction and loss of range of motion (Fig. 1–10).

Some of the aspiration and arthrographic techniques that may be used in the assessment of prosthetic joints are discussed in the subsequent paragraphs.

HIP ASPIRATION

When aspiration of the hip is to be performed, the patient is placed in a supine position on the fluoroscopy table with the hip in question closest to the person performing the procedure. The skin overlying the greater trochanter is marked and subsequently prepped and draped in sterile fashion. A 10-ml solution containing 8 ml lidocaine HCl 1% (10 mg/ml) (Abbott Laboratories, North Chicago, IL) mixed with 2 ml 8.4% solution of sodium bicarbonate (American Pharmaceutical Partners, Los Angeles, CA) is used to anesthetize the skin and subcutaneous tissue. From an anterolateral approach, a 20-gauge, 3½-inch spinal needle (Becton Dickinson, Franklin Lakes, NJ) is introduced until contact with the prosthetic femoral neck is made. The anterolateral approach is taken so that the tip of the needle can be visualized at all times; this is similar to the straight lateral approach over the greater trochanter that is advocated by others. The stylet is removed and aspiration with a sterile syringe is performed. Occasionally, repositioning of the needle tip is required in order to obtain an adequate sample of fluid. This can be accomplished by "walking" the tip across the femoral neck, being mindful of femoral vessels and nerves medially. If this fails to yield any fluid, one may instill, under fluoroscopic guidance, 5 ml of ionic contrast such as diatrizoate meglumine 60% (Reno-M-60;

Bracco Diagnostic, Princeton, NJ) or nonionic contrast such as iopamidol (Isovue-M-200; Bracco Diagnostics, Princeton, NJ) if the patient has a history of contrast allergy. This allows the intra-articular position of the spinal needle to be confirmed. Some of the contrast solution is reaspirated and sent for culture, sensitivities, and Gram stain. Images are obtained for documentation. It is also possible to use 5 ml of sterile saline for reaspiration, but needle tip position cannot be reliably confirmed under fluoroscopy when this solution is used. Lidocaine should not be utilized to obtain joint fluid samples, as it is bacteriostatic; iodinated contrast can be used if the specimen is processed within 3 hours of acquisition.[15]

Girdlestone Hip Aspiration

To perform a Girdlestone hip aspiration, the skin overlying the affected hip is prepped and draped in the usual sterile fashion, and 8 ml of lidocaine HCl 1% solution mixed with 2 ml of 8.4% sodium bicarbonate solution is used as a local anesthetic for the skin and underlying subcutaneous tissue only. A 20-gauge 3½-inch spinal needle is then introduced using an anterolateral approach. The tip of the needle is directed toward a point just above the approximate midpoint of a line drawn between the greater and lesser trochanters (Fig. 1–11).[16] A sterile syringe directly attached to the spinal needle is used to aspirate the joint fluid. Spot films centered over the hip are obtained to demonstrate tip position prior to the conclusion of the study.

HIP ARTHROGRAPHY

Arthrography of prosthetic hips may be performed after aspiration of joint fluid. With the 20-gauge 3½-inch spinal needle in place, 15 to 25 ml of iodinated contrast

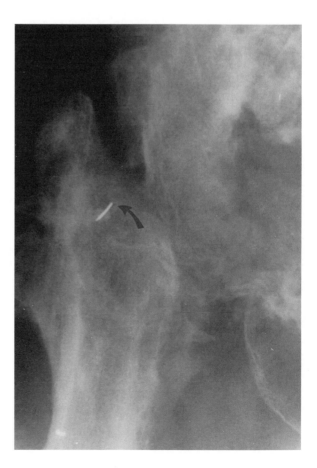

FIGURE 1–11 An AP view of a Girdlestone hip with the tip of a needle (arrow) that was used for local skin and subcutaneous anesthesia demonstrates where a separate needle used for aspiration should be positioned. The tip of a 20-gauge 3½-inch spinal needle is positioned at a point halfway between the greater and lesser trochanters, where aspiration is attempted.

is injected via an extension tube that is connected to the hub of the needle. An AP scout image of the hip, including the distal femoral tip, should be obtained prior to the injection of any contrast so it can serve as a baseline image.

After administration of the contrast under fluoroscopic control, stress maneuvers are performed on the hip. A radiograph of the hip is obtained while pushing on the patient's leg, driving the femoral head craniad. This is followed by a spot film of the hip while distracting or pulling forces are applied on the leg (Fig. 1–12). The various arthrographic signs of loosening previously described may be found. Not uncommonly, lymphatic opacification is encountered; this should not necessarily be interpreted as loosening, as it may also be seen in synovitis and in overdistension of the joint by fluid. The contrast is reaspirated via the indwelling needle at the conclusion of the study.

Lidocaine or Steroid Challenge

In the preoperative assessment of native hip pain, administration of intra-articular anesthetic with or without a longer-acting steroid solution may help to determine whether the patient's symptoms originate in the hip or are referred. The technique is identical to that of a hip aspiration except that the tip of the spinal needle is confirmed to be intra-articular by injecting a small amount (~3 ml) of iodinated contrast through an attached extension tube and following that with either 7 to 10 ml of an intermediate-acting anesthetic alone, such as Sensorcaine 0.5% (bupivacaine), *or* 10 ml of a solution of 7 to 8 ml of Sensorcaine 0.5% premixed with a steroid solution such as Depo-Medrol 80 (methylprednisolone acetate suspension, 80 mg/L; Pharmacia & Upjohn, Kalamazoo, MI), or with 2.5 ml of Celestone Soluspan (betamethasone sodium phosphate and betamethasone acetate, 6 mg/ml; Schering, Kenilworth, NJ).

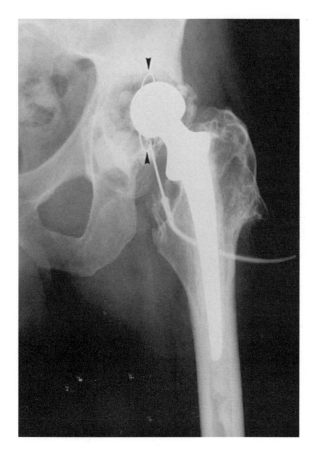

FIGURE 1–12 Dynamic images of a total hip arthroplasty using the push-pull technique. A shift in the acetabular component (arrowheads) is demonstrated when a driving force is applied to the hip.

KNEE ASPIRATION AND ARTHROGRAPHY

After sterile preparation and drape of the anterior aspect of the knee, 8 to 9 ml of lidocaine HCl 1% solution mixed with 1 to 2 ml of 8.4% sodium bicarbonate solution is given to anesthetize the skin and subcutaneous tissue overlying the medial aspect of the patellofemoral joint. A 22-gauge, 1½-inch needle is then introduced into the joint space from the superomedial aspect of the patella, and fluid is aspirated. The fluid is generally sent for routine aerobic and anaerobic culture and sensitivity, Gram stain, and cell count. A superolateral approach may be attempted if the medial approach is unsuccessful, although the distance along the lateral facet is believed to be longer.

Arthrographic assessment of the joint is performed by attaching extension tubing to the end of the 22-gauge needle and administering at least 20 ml of iodinated contrast through the tubing. Prior to administration of the contrast, scout views of the knee should be obtained to provide baseline images. After moving the knee through passive range of motion, an AP image of the knee with the tibial tray in tangent and a lateral view of the prosthesis in profile should be obtained to assess for wear of the prosthetic liner and to check for loosening (Fig. 1–13). The patient is then asked to walk for several minutes before additional overhead AP, lateral, and patellar views are obtained. This exercise and weightbearing theoretically allows the contrast to flow into potential areas of loosening.

SHOULDER ARTHROGRAPHY

Arthrography of a postarthroplasty shoulder is not commonly performed, although the approach would be similar to arthrography of a native shoulder. The patient is placed supine on the fluoroscopy table, and the anterior aspect of the affected shoulder is prepped and draped in the usual sterile fashion. Local anesthetic—8 ml of lidocaine HCl 1% and 2 ml of 8.4% sodium bicarbonate solution—is applied. A 22-gauge 3½-inch spinal needle is introduced, using an anterior approach, into the glenohumeral joint, typically at the junction of the middle and inferior thirds of the humeral head as it articulates with the glenoid. For tip position and arthrography, 10 to 15 ml of contrast are used, and scout and postcontrast AP and axillary images of the shoulder are obtained (Fig. 1–14).

Computed Tomography

Computed tomography (CT) is better than conventional radiography because of its high resolution, its transaxial and image-reformatting capabilities, and its superior spatial resolution.[17, 18] However, artifacts such as beam hardening, partial volume effects, scatter, and misregistration of data (or aliasing) have placed limitations on its utility in the past. As CT hardware and image reformatting software have improved, some of these imaging artifacts have been minimized or circumvented.[19, 20] Imaging strategies such as utilizing smaller cross-sectional images of orthopaedic appliances help to diminish the x-ray attenuation responsible for some of the missing projection data in image reconstruction,[19] and using high-frequency filters and increasing the window width in image reconstruction have helped to improve the assessment of a joint that has undergone arthroplasty.[21] Likewise, advances in orthopaedic hardware and the use of materials with lower x-ray attenuation coefficients, such as titanium, help to decrease missing projection data that cause beam-hardening artifacts in the presence of such materials as stainless steel and cobalt-chrome alloys.[19] However, Wetzner and colleagues state that the efficacy of CT has yet to be determined.[22]

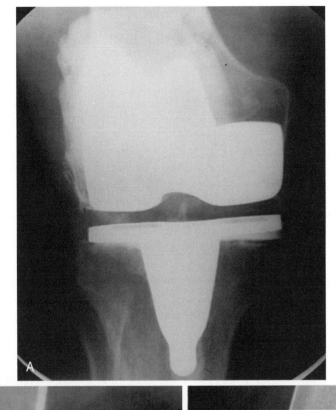

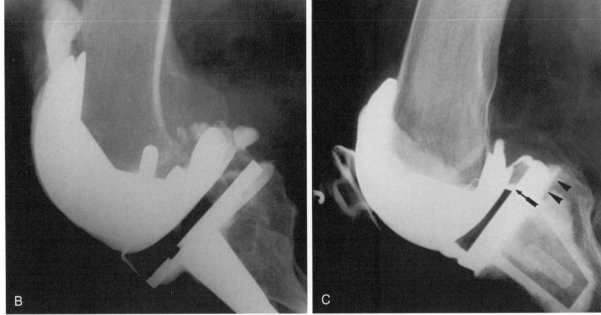

FIGURE 1–13 A: An AP view of a total knee arthroplasty during routine arthrography. **B:** A lateral view of a total knee arthroplasty during arthroplasty. The femoral condylar components should be superimposed on each other. The liner should be assessed in profile. **C:** A lateral view of a total knee arthrogram of another patient that highlights some normal variants seen during arthrography. Some prosthetic liners show filling of a linear cleft, which is normal (arrow). It occurs because a cutout has been made for the posterior cruciate ligament. Likewise, it is not uncommon for contrast to undermine the tibial tray without causing infection or loosening (arrowheads).

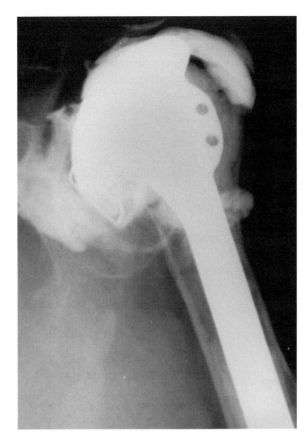

FIGURE 1–14 An arthrogram of a shoulder demonstrates contrast outlining the subacromial subdeltoid bursa, suggesting a rotator cuff tear.

PREOPERATIVE CT

In the setting of trauma, CT may be helpful in assessing affected joints; it can be used to evaluate the congruence of articulating surfaces, to look for intra-articular loose bodies, to determine the presence and types of fractures, and to investigate soft-tissue abnormalities.[22, 23] Likewise, in the evaluation of certain arthritides and congenital abnormalities, such as dislocation of the hip, CT has proven useful for defining complex anatomic relationships and disruptions and for planning the placement and sizing of a particular prosthetic device.[23–26]

CT arthrography can be performed like routine arthrography and is useful to assess cartilage and detect loose bodies. It utilizes the double contrast effect of air instilled into the joint space with several ml of contrast to outline the articular surface within the joint. The joint is prepped and draped in the usual sterile fashion. A 22-gauge 3½-inch spinal needle (for the shoulder) or a 20-gauge 3½-inch spinal needle (for the hip) is advanced into the joint after administration of skin and subcutaneous local anesthetic. The inner surface of the joint is coated with 3 to 5 ml of contrast. We instill 0.3 ml of epinephrine 1:1000 solution with the contrast to delay absorption of the contrast. This is followed by 8 to 10 ml of air, which is administered via an extension tube attached to the indwelling spinal needle. This allows for distension of the joint and for the double contrast effect of air outlining the radiodense contrast. The joint is imaged by CT using thin axial sections.

POSTOPERATIVE CT

In the past, conventional tomography had been considered the best means of evaluating the postarthroplasty joint. However, despite the occurrence of the artifacts previously mentioned, CT, with its ability to produce reformatted images in the orthogonal plane, allows better resolution of the edges and interfaces and provides more detailed information about surrounding soft tissues, muscles, fascial planes, and fluid collections (abscesses, hematomas) than does conventional tomography.[19] Reformatting the images on other planes does not require that the patient receive additional radiation, as would be necessary in conventional tomography, should orthogonal images be desired.[19]

Various authors state that CT may be useful for assessing bone stock in those being considered for revision arthroplasty and for detecting abnormalities on the contralateral side such as avascular necrosis.[19, 22] Mian and colleagues describe the utility of CT when measuring acetabular cup anteversion and retroversion in a patient with a dislocating total hip prosthesis; the angle of the cup is measured on the CT display console.[27]

Complications of arthroplasty may be determined more precisely by using CT. The presence and location of heterotopic ossification and cement, soft-tissue abscesses and fluid collections, and areas of osteolysis can be pinpointed by CT (Fig. 1–15).[19, 22, 27]

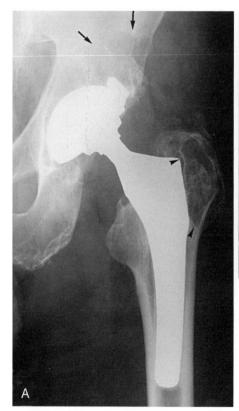

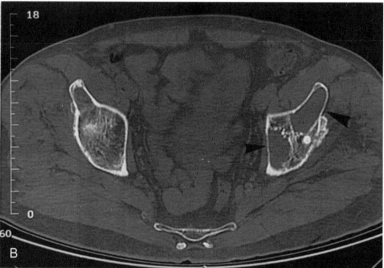

FIGURE 1–15 A: An AP view of a left hip demonstrates areas of osteolysis involving the acetabulum (arrows) and greater trochanter (arrowheads). **B:** An axial CT image through the acetabula demonstrates the osteolysis seen on the plain radiograph; CT images are also useful to assess residual bone stock, fractures, and soft-tissue abnormalities.

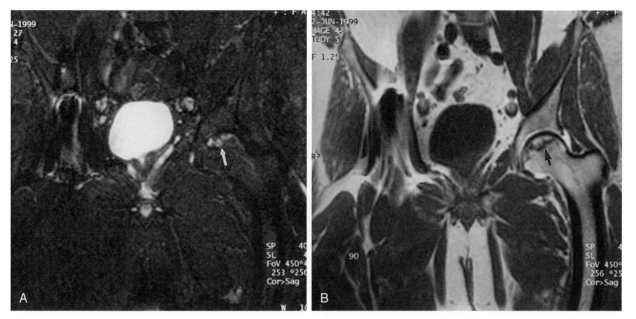

FIGURE 1–16 A: A coronal T1-weighted image of both hips in a 36-year-old male with a history of Crohn's disease. Note the artifact on the right, which is related to a hip arthroplasty. The native left hip is abnormal and has a geographic area demarcated by a rim that shows low signal intensity along the femoral head (arrow). **B:** There is high signal intensity (arrow) on T2-weighted sequences, which is indicative of osteonecrosis.

Magnetic Resonance Imaging

Because of marked susceptibility to artifacts produced by prostheses, magnetic resonance imaging (MRI) is of limited use in the assessment of postimplant joints. Like CT, MRI may be most valuable in the assessment of complications in a native contralateral joint and in the soft tissues outside the area of distortion caused by the prosthesis (Fig. 1–16). Its inherent soft-tissue contrast, oblique imaging plane capabilities, and lack of ionizing radiation are potential benefits of this modality for the patient.

Summary

A variety of diagnostic and therapeutic imaging strategies and interventions are available to the orthopaedic surgeon and radiologist for managing joint arthroplasties. We have described how to perform some minimally invasive procedures such as arthrography using a specific imaging modality and therapeutic joint injections, demonstrated some postarthroplasty complications, and provided an overview of standard images obtained in the pre- and postoperative patient so as to help others to recognize the normal appearances of arthroplasties and their complications and normal variants and to understand some of the uses and limitations of the technology available.

REFERENCES

1. Coventry MB, Beckenbaugh RD, Nolan DR, et al. Total hip arthroplasties: a study of postoperative course and early complications. J Bone Joint Surg Am 1974;56:273.
2. Kavanaugh BF, Dewitz MA, Ilsrup DM, et al. Charnley total hip arthroplasty with cement, fifteen-year results. J Bone Joint Surg Am 1989;71:1496–1503.

3. Sculco TP. Primary total knee replacement. In Petty W, ed. Total Joint Replacement. Philadelphia: WB Saunders, 1991, pp. 507–531.

4. Tigges S, Stiles RG, Meli RJ, et al. Hip aspiration: a cost-effective and accurate method of evaluating the potentially infected hip prosthesis. Radiology 1993;189:485–488.

5. Long BW, Rafert JA. The Pelvis and Hip Joint. In Long BW, Rafert JA, eds. Orthopaedic Radiography. Philadelphia: WB Saunders, 1995, pp. 308–313.

6. Gold RH, Nasser S, Stall SM. Conventional roentgenography with special techniques for follow-up hip arthroplasty. In Amstutz HC, ed. Hip Arthroplasty. New York: Churchill Livingstone, 1991, pp. 121–170.

7. Clarke IC, Gruen T, Matos M, et al. Improved methods for quantitative radiographic evaluation with particular reference to total hip arthroplasty. Clin Orthop 1976;121:83.

8. Baldursson H, Hansson LI, Olsson TH, et al. Migration of the acetabular socket after total hip replacement determined by roentgen stereophotogrammetry. Acta Orthop Scand 1980;51:535.

9. Amstutz HC, Ouzounian T, Grauer D, et al. The grid radiograph: a simple technique for consistent high-resolution visualization of the hip. J Bone Joint Surg Am 1986;68:1052.

10. Freedman MT. Radiologic aspects of femoral head replacements and cup mold arthroplasties. Radiol Clin North Am 1975;13:45–56.

11. Allen AM, Ward WG, Pope TL Jr. Imaging of the total knee arthroplasty. Radiol Clin North Am 1995;33:289–303.

12. Figgie HE III, Goldberg VM, Heiple KG, et al. The influence of tibial-patellofemoral location on function of the knee in patients with the posterior stabilized condylar knee prosthesis. J Bone Joint Surg Am 1986;68:1035–1040.

13. Slivka J, Resnick D. An improved radiographic view of the glenohumeral joint. J Can Assoc Radiol 1979;30:83–85.

14. Slawson SH, Everson LI, Craig EV. The radiology of total shoulder replacement. Radiol Clin North Am 1995;33:305–318.

15. Dory MA, Wautelet MJ. Arthroscopy in septic arthritis: lidocaine- and iodine-containing contrast media are bacteriostatic. Arthritis Rheum 1985;28:198–203.

16. Swan JS, Braunstein EM, Capello W. Aspiration of the hip in patients treated with Girdlestone arthroplasty. AJR Am J Roentgenol 1991;156:545–546.

17. Amstutz H. Dysplasia and congenital dislocation of the hip. In Amstutz HC, ed. Hip Arthroplasty. New York: Churchill Livingstone, 1992, p. 723.

18. Vannier M, Totty W, Stevens W, et al. Musculoskeletal applications of three-dimensional surface reconstructions. Orthop Clin North Am 1985;16:543.

19. Robertson DD, Magid D, Poss R, et al. Enhanced computed tomographic techniques for the evaluation of total hip arthroplasty. J Arthroplasty 1989;4:271–276.

20. Robertson DD, Weiss PJ, Fishman EK, et al. Evaluation of CT techniques for reducing artifact in the presence of metallic orthopedic implants. J Comput Assist Tomogr 1988;12:236.

21. Egund N, Pettersson H, Frost S, et al. The potential of computed tomography in visualising structures inside the metal cup in surface-replacement total hip arthroplasty. Skeletal Radiol 1987;16:201–204.

22. Wetzner SM, Newberg AH, McKenzie JD. Radiographic evaluation of symptomatic hip arthroplasty. In Turner RH, Scheller AD, eds. Revision Total Hip Arthroplasty. New York: Grune & Stratton, 1982, pp. 44–47.

23. Dias JJ, Johnson GV, Finlay DBL, et al. Preoperative evaluation for uncemented hip arthroplasty: the role of computerised tomography. J Bone Joint Surg Br 1989;71B:43–46.

24. Green A, Norris TR. Imaging techniques for glenohumeral arthritis and glenohumeral arthroplasty. Clin Orthop 1994;307:7–17.

25. Xenakis TA, Gelalis ID, Koukoubis TD, et al. Neglected congenital dislocation of the hip. Role of computed tomography and computer-aided design for total hip arthroplasty. J Arthroplasty 1996;11:893–898.

26. Mathis KB, Noble PC, Tullos HS. Preoperative templating in revision total hip arthroplasty. In Bono JV, McCarthy JC, Thornhill TS, et al., eds. Revision Total Hip Arthroplasty. New York: Springer-Verlag, 1999, pp. 129–134.

27. Mian SW, Truchly G, Pflum FA. Computed tomography measurement of acetabular cup anteversion and retroversion in total hip arthroplasty. Clin Orthop 1992;276:206–209.

2

Orthopaedic Implants of the Elbow, Wrist, and Hand

PETER J. L. JEBSON

DEAN S. LOUIS

Copyright © 2001 by Peter J. L. Jebson and Dean S. Louis, illustrations only included in this chapter.

Elbow

Total elbow arthroplasty is most commonly performed in patients with advanced rheumatoid arthritis that is refractory to medical management. Implant arthroplasty of the elbow is also indicated in patients with complex fractures or nonunions of the distal humerus and posttraumatic or primary degenerative arthritis of the elbow joint.

Numerous implant designs have been used. There are three basic design types that differ in the degree of inherent stability provided by the prosthesis itself:

1. A nonconstrained, or resurfacing, device (Fig. 2–1) that consists of two separate metal components that articulate by means of a high-density polyethylene component;

2. A semiconstrained device that is hinged but provides some lateral motion (Fig. 2–2);

3. A constrained device that is constructed of separate ulnar and humeral components that are hinged by a bushing (Fig. 2–3).

The constrained prostheses consist of rigid hinges that result in significant stress transfer to the adjacent bone/cement interface and subsequent osteolysis and implant loosening (see Fig. 2–3). The nonconstrained, or resurfacing, devices were introduced to alleviate the loosening problems but are associated with implant subluxation and dislocation. The semiconstrained devices (see Fig. 2–2) improve joint stability with minimization of stress transfer to the adjacent bone/cement interface.

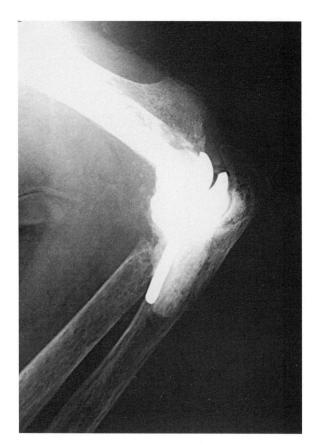

FIGURE 2–1   A lateral radiograph of a cemented, nonconstrained, or resurfacing, implant in which the absence of the surgically resected radial head may be noted.

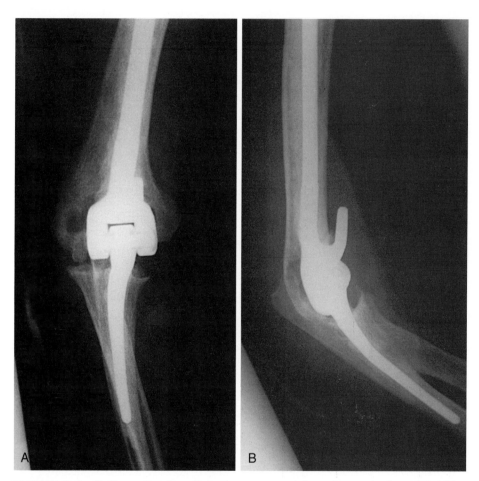

FIGURE 2–2   Radiographs of an elbow show a cemented, semiconstrained, modified Morrey-Coonrad prosthesis. **A:** An AP view demonstrates the valgus alignment of the prosthesis. **B:** A lateral view best demonstrates an anterior flange on the humeral component. A bone block taken from the resected trochlea is usually inserted between the humeral shaft and the flange to enhance the fixation and stability of the implant. Early osteolysis of the lateral humeral condyle without implant loosening is apparent.

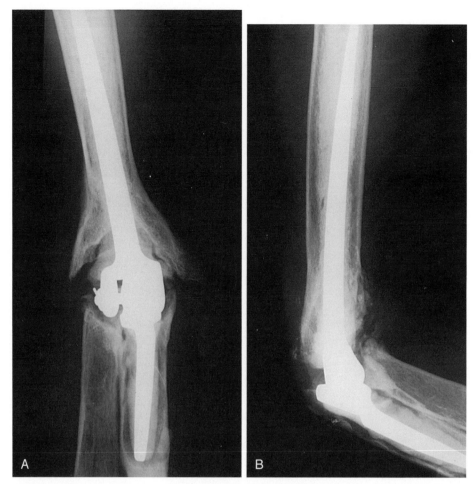

FIGURE 2–3 A and **B:** Osteolysis can be particularly severe, as is illustrated in these views of a constrained elbow prosthesis. Extensive osteolysis, loosening of the ulnar component, remodeling of the proximal ulna, and thinning of the adjacent cortices may be seen. Infection should always be ruled out in a patient with osteolysis and a loose implant arthroplasty.

Wrist

Arthrodesis of the wrist is most commonly indicated for patients with symptomatic rheumatoid, degenerative, or posttraumatic arthritis involving the radiocarpal and midcarpal articulations. There are several techniques for achieving wrist arthrodesis. Early fixation methods involved a single or multiple pins, wires, or rods that were placed down a metacarpal shaft (usually the index or long metacarpal) or through the intermetacarpal spaces. Figure 2–4 demonstrates the single-rod technique. Note the solid, well-consolidated fusion mass and the broken rod (a common complication) that was inserted down the third metacarpal shaft, across the carpus, and into the radial shaft. Figure 2–5 illustrates the dual-rod technique, in which two Steinman pins are inserted in the second and third intermetacarpal spaces. The simultaneous resection of the distal ulna may be noted. More recently, wrist arthrodesis has involved immediate rigid fixation utilizing dorsal plating (Fig. 2–6). The plate is usually applied along, and secured to, the shafts of the third metacarpal and radius. Alternatively, if the midcarpal space is well preserved, a radiocarpal arthrodesis may be performed. Figure 2–7 is the posteroanterior (PA) view of the wrist of a young man who underwent a radiolunate arthrodesis for persistent posttraumatic ulnar translocation instability of the carpus. An external fixator has been applied to the index metacarpal and radial shafts. The radial styloid fracture was fixed with three

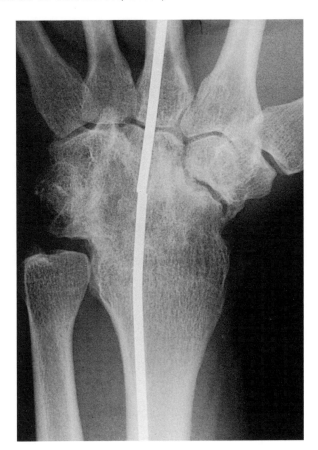

FIGURE 2–4 A single-rod wrist arthrodesis with fatigue failure of the rod. The intramedullary rod has been inserted along the third metacarpal shaft, across the carpus, and into the radial shaft.

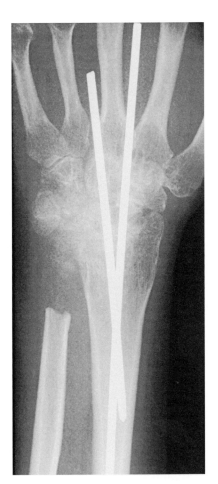

FIGURE 2–5 A dual-rod wrist arthrodesis uses two Steinmann pins.

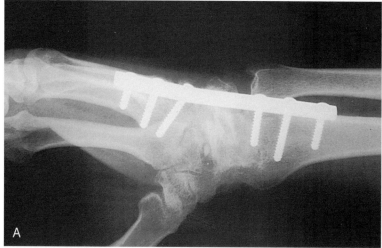

FIGURE 2–6 **A** and **B:** Two views of a wrist arthrodesis performed with dorsal plating.

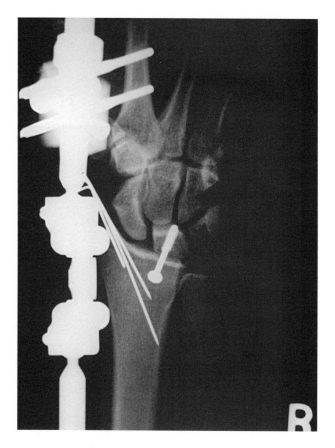

FIGURE 2–7 An AP view of a radiolunate arthrodesis demonstrates the use of an external fixator and a partially threaded interfragmentary screw.

smooth Kirschner wires. The radiolunate arthrodesis was performed with a partially threaded interfragmentary screw.

Hand

A variety of silicone implants have been used in the upper extremity. The implants were designed to replace specific excised structures, such as the distal ulna, the carpus, and the metacarpophalangeal (MCP) and interphalangeal joints. Silicone implant arthroplasty used to be indicated in patients with various degenerative, posttraumatic, and inflammatory arthritic conditions. However, because of the significant complications of implant fracture, dislocation, and fragmentation with particulate reactive silicone synovitis, their use is now limited to the MCP joints of patients with advanced, functionally limiting inflammatory arthritis. Carpal bone, radial head, and distal ulnar silicone replacements are no longer available. The concept of replacing a specific bone or joint with an artificial implant has continued with the design and introduction of a variety of metallic prostheses. These implants, however, have also fallen into disfavor because of instability, loosening, and dislocation of the implant (Figs. 2–8 through 2–16).

Text continued on page 32

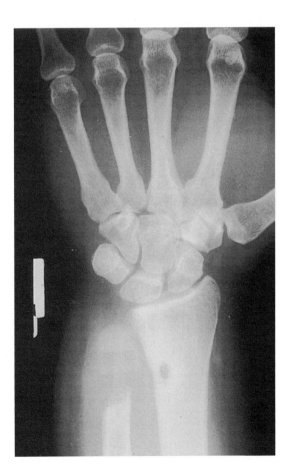

FIGURE 2–8 On this AP view of the wrist, the resection of the distal ulna and the silicone cap replacement may be seen.

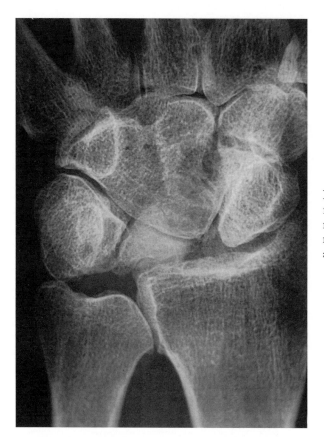

FIGURE 2–9 A capitohamate arthrodesis has been performed in conjunction with resection of the lunate and its replacement by a silicone implant in this patient with avascular necrosis of the lunate (Kienböck's disease). The compressed appearance of the implant is visible.

FIGURE 2–10 An oblique view of the thumb illustrates fragmentation of a trapezial silicone implant. This replacement was performed because of osteoarthritis of the trapeziometacarpal joint.

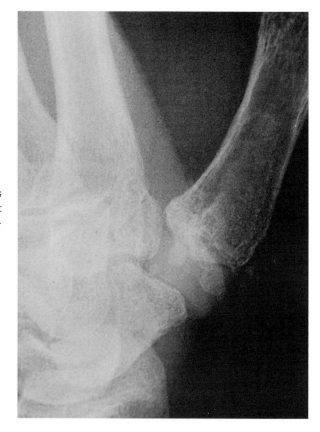

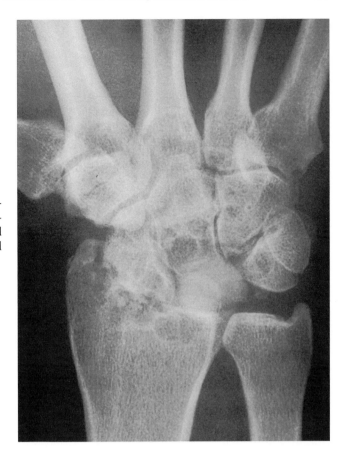

FIGURE 2–11 An AP view of a wrist with classic silicone synovitis associated with a silicone implant arthroplasty of the lunate. Destruction of the radioscaphoid articulation, erosions and subchondral cysts in the distal radius, and the adjacent carpal bones may be seen.

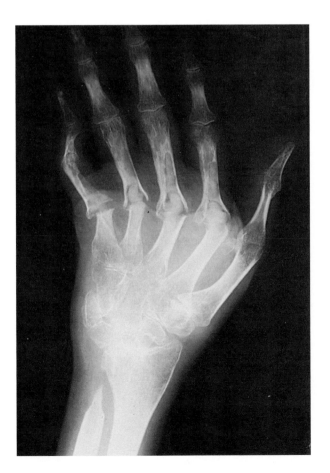

FIGURE 2–12 An AP view of the wrist of a patient with rheumatoid arthritis who underwent resection of the distal ulna and replacement of the MCP joints with hinged silicone prostheses. Recurrent ulnar drift of the fingers has resulted in implant fracture and dislocation.

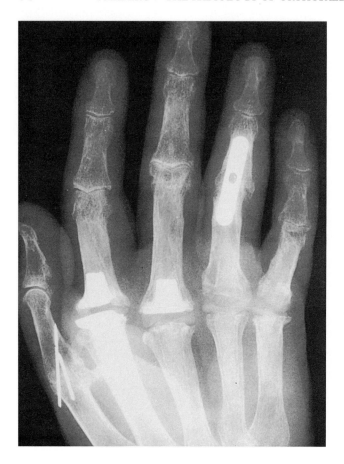

FIGURE 2–13   In this view, it can be seen that metallic sleeves called grommets have been inserted for protection of the silicone implants because of concerns regarding accelerated implant wear by the adjacent surfaces of the metacarpal and proximal phalangeal shafts. This patient has also undergone an arthrodesis of the MCP joint of the thumb that uses two Kirschner wires and an arthrodesis of the proximal interphalangeal joint of the ring finger that uses a mini fragment plate and screws.

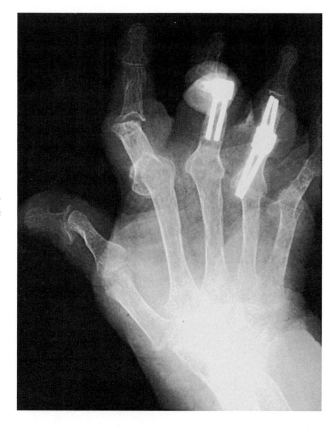

FIGURE 2–14   Hinged metallic implants in proximal interphalangeal joints may be seen in a patient with severe erosive rheumatoid arthritis.

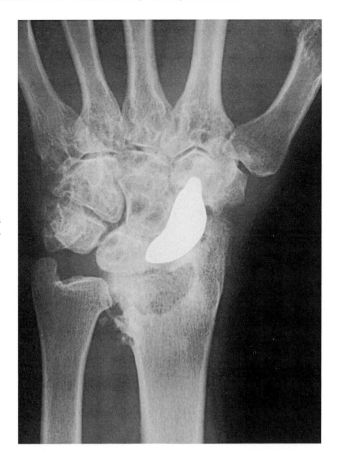

FIGURE 2–15 A titanium scaphoid implant has been used to replace a silicone implant because of reactive silicone synovitis.

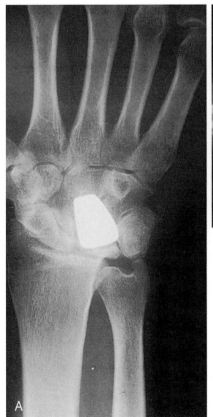

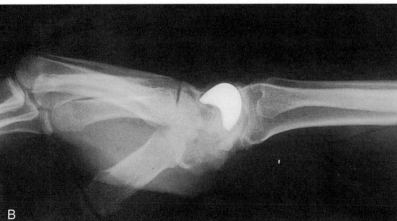

FIGURE 2–16 **A:** A titanium lunate implant has been performed in a patient with Kienböck's disease. **B:** The implant has undergone palmar flexion and has eroded into the dorsal aspect of the capitate.

Fractures of the hand and wrist may be stabilized by a variety of implants including wires, screws, plates, and external fixators, or a combination of devices. Implant selection is based upon several factors including which bone is involved, the fracture pattern, and associated injuries (Figs. 2–17 through 2–26).

Text continued on page 37

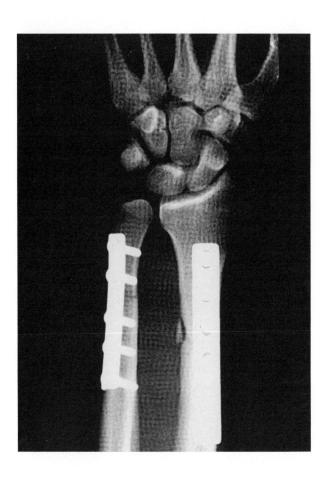

FIGURE 2–17 Fractures of the radial and ulnar shafts have been anatomically reduced and internally fixed with plates and screws.

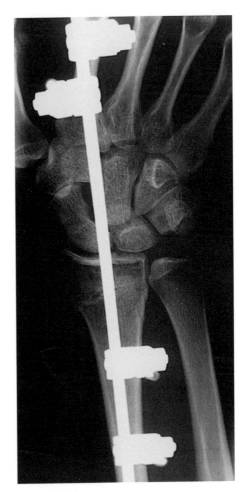

FIGURE 2–18 Fractures of the distal radius may be stabilized by using an external fixator. There are a variety of commercially available external fixators, but all have the common feature of pin placement in the index metacarpal and proximal radial shafts. This particular fixator is composed of a single metal bar connected to the fixator pins by clamps.

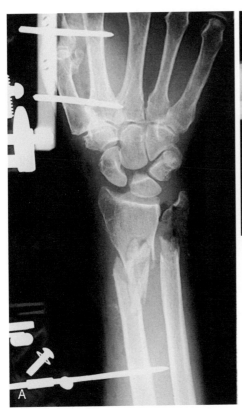

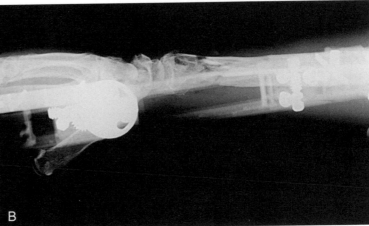

FIGURE 2–19 **A:** This external fixator has a unique gear mechanism that permits precise manipulation of the fracture. **B:** A radiolucent frame permits visualization of the fracture's alignment on the lateral radiographic image.

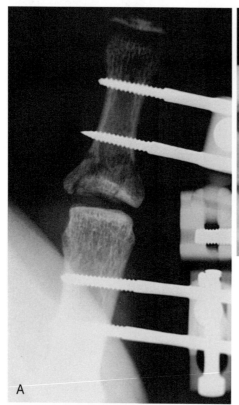

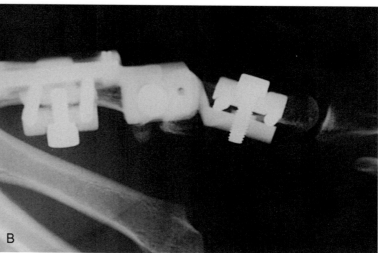

FIGURE 2–20   A: The principle of external fixation of the fracture of a long bone has also been applied to certain fractures of the smaller tubular bones of the hand. These devices are referred to as mini external fixators and, as is the case with their larger counterparts, many different types exist. **B:** The particular device used in this patient, who suffered a comminuted intra-articular fracture of the proximal phalanx of the thumb, is composed of a nonradiolucent frame and ball hinge articulation.

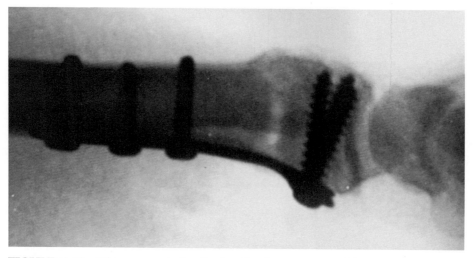

FIGURE 2–21   This extra-articular distal radius fracture was stabilized with a plate and screws that were applied along the volar cortex of the radius.

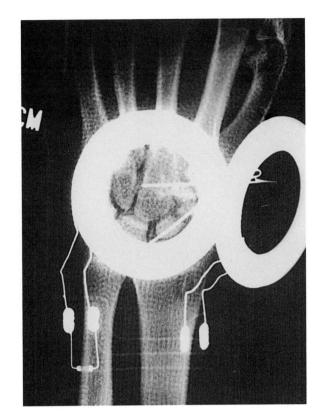

FIGURE 2–22 The scaphoid and capitate fractures in this patient were stabilized with Kirschner wires. The radiodense circular structures and connecting wires are components of a bone stimulator that is applied directly over a fracture or site of nonunion to enhance bony healing.

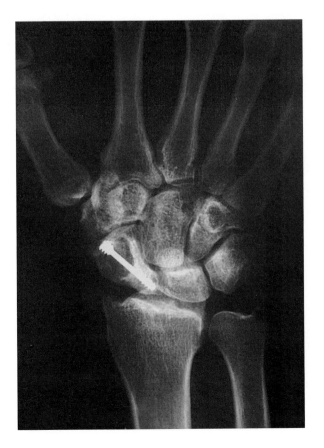

FIGURE 2–23 The scaphoid nonunion and early degenerative arthritis in this patient were treated by excision of the radial styloid and internal fixation of the scaphoid with a single screw. The design of this screw includes the presence of a different pitch between the screw threads at either end, which provides compression as the screw is inserted.

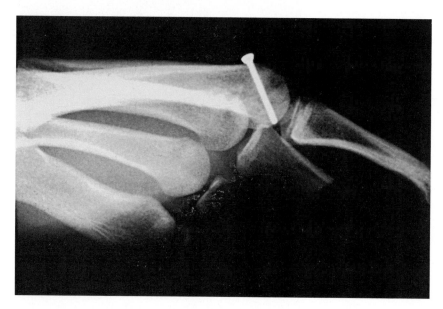

FIGURE 2–24 This open reduction and internal fixation of a fracture of a metacarpal head was performed with an interfragmentary screw of alternative design.

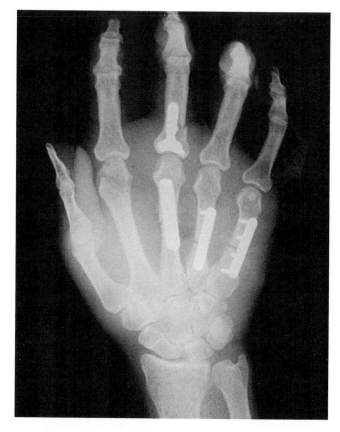

FIGURE 2–25 This internal fixation of multiple fractures of the metacarpal and phalangeal shaft uses mini plates and screws.

FIGURE 2–26 A lateral radiograph of a digit illustrates a bone anchor that has migrated into the pulp space of the fingertip. Bone anchors, which are used to reattach avulsed tendons, ligaments, or joint capsules, may have a variety of designs. The anchor seen in this figure was used to attach the terminal slip of the digital extensor tendon.

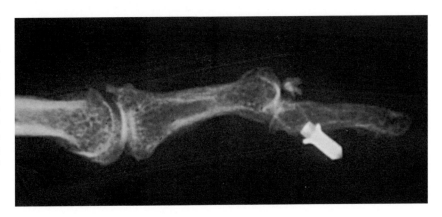

BIBLIOGRAPHY

Adams BD, Frykman GK, Taleisnik J. Treatment of scaphoid non-union with casting and pulsed electromagnetic fields: a study continuation. J Hand Surg 1992;17A:910–914.

Berger RA, Beckenbaugh RD, Linscheid RI. Arthroplasty of the hand and wrist. In Green DP, Hotchkiss RN, Pederson WC, eds. Green's Operative Hand Surgery, 4th ed. Philadelphia: Churchill-Livingstone, 1999, pp. 147–151.

Cooney WP. External fixation of distal radius fractures. Clin Orthop 1983;180:44–49.

Ewald FC, Simmons ED, Sullivan JA, et al. Capitellocondylar total elbow replacement in rheumatoid arthritis: long-term results. J Bone Joint Surg 1993;75A:498–507.

Hastings HH. Wrist arthrodesis. In Green DP, Hotchkiss RN, Pederson WC, eds. Green's Operative Hand Surgery, 4th ed. Philadelphia: Churchill-Livingstone, 1999, pp.131–146.

Herbert TJ, Fischer WE. Management of the fractured scaphoid using a new bone screw. J Bone Joint Surg 1984;66B:114–123.

Morrey BF, Adams RA. Semiconstrained elbow replacement for rheumatoid arthritis. J Bone Joint Surg 1992;74A:479.

Stern PJ. Fractures of the metacarpals and phalanges. In Green DP, Hotchkiss RN, Pederson WC, eds. Green's Operative Hand Surgery, 4th ed. Philadelphia: Churchill-Livingstone, 1999, pp. 711–771.

3

—

Trauma

DAVID J. HAK

—

Many minor or stable fractures may be treated nonoperatively, but a large number of fractures are now treated operatively with a wide variety of internal and external fixation devices. Radiographic examination after fracture fixation is necessary to evaluate the fracture's healing. When healing fails to occur, radiographs may reveal loss of fixation, with hardware failure or migration.

Adjacent visualized regions should also be carefully inspected in the event that additional fractures are present that were not initially apparent. It is especially important to carefully evaluate the femoral neck in patients with femoral shaft fractures because associated ipsilateral femoral neck fractures occur in 2 to 6% of cases. Many of these femoral neck fractures are nondisplaced and may be initially missed in up to 11% of the cases.

External Fixation

External fixation devices consist of pins or wires that are placed percutaneously into the bone above and below a fracture site. These pins or wires are connected by various clamps to external fixation rods or rings. There are three basic types of external fixators: standard pin fixators, ring fixators, and hybrid fixators.

External fixation is commonly used for open fractures that have significant associated soft-tissue injuries. In addition to stabilizing the fracture, it also permits local wound care to be performed. External fixation may also be chosen for the management of closed fractures in cases in which an acceptable closed reduction of the fracture can be achieved. Stabilization with the external fixator maintains the reduction, resisting the deforming forces caused by muscular contraction. The use of an external fixator may eliminate the need for further surgical dissection and the associated devascularization that can impede fracture healing (Figs. 3–1 through 3–3).

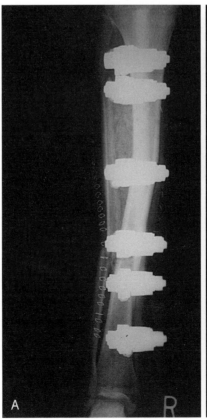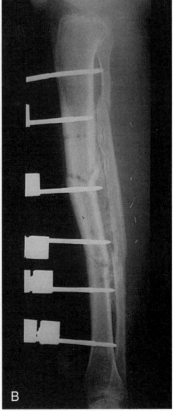

FIGURE 3–1 A: Uniplanar fixation is the simplest form of external fixation. This open, segmental tibial shaft fracture has been treated by using a uniplanar standard pin external fixator. Two pins have been placed percutaneously into each segment and connected to an external rod by clamps. In this case, the external fixation rod is made of a radiolucent carbon fiber composite to optimize subsequent radiographic imaging. In this AP view, skin staples are present because subsequent bone grafting was performed to stimulate fracture healing. **B:** A lateral view shows the fracture's alignment. The x-ray has cut off parts of the clamps and external rods. The posterolateral bone graft has been placed along the interosseous membrane between the fibula and tibia. The vascular clips were placed when a gastrocnemius rotational flap was performed to achieve soft-tissue coverage of the open fracture site.

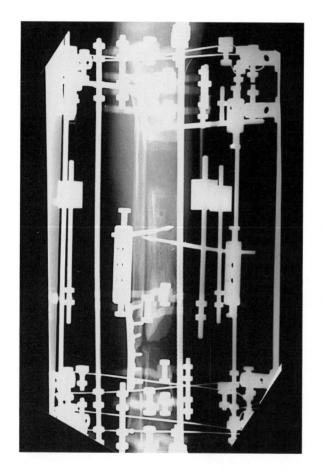

FIGURE 3–2   Ring fixators utilize thin wires under tension that are attached to a circular or semicircular ring. The Ilizarov technique refers to a specific method of lengthening bone by using a corticotomy and gradual distraction, but the term *Ilizarov fixator* is commonly applied to any form of ring fixator. The patient in this figure sustained an open tibial fracture and had segmental bone loss at the middle and distal junctions. A corticotomy was performed inferior to the tibial tubercle and was followed by gradual distraction of the intervening segment at a rate of 1 mm per day. Early consolidation is seen in this newly regenerated bone.

FIGURE 3–3 The combination of a ring fixator and a standard pin fixator is referred to as a hybrid external fixator. This type of fixator is commonly used in fractures involving the proximal or distal tibia. **A:** In this AP view of the ankle, cannulated screws have been placed across the major fracture line that extends into the ankle joint. The tensioned thin wires below these screws are parallel to the ankle joint. **B:** A lateral view of the tibia shows the distal fixation ring and clamps. The ring is attached to a uniplanar rod connected to the two standard pins in the proximal tibial shaft (located anteriorly but cut off by the x-ray collimation).

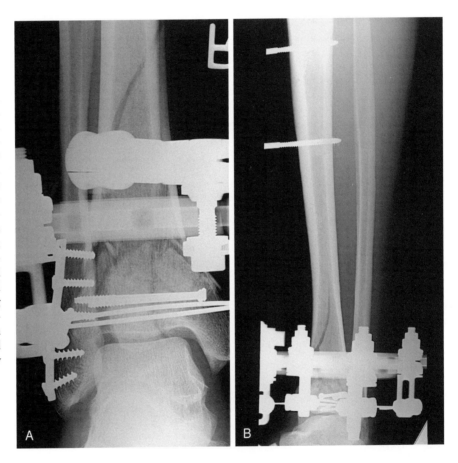

Internal Fixation

A myriad of internal fixation devices are available for fracture fixation. Narrow-diameter trocar-tipped wires called Kirschner wires, or k-wires, are commonly utilized to secure small fracture fragments. These wires may be placed internally or percutaneously. Because they are smooth, they do not provide interfragmentary compression and can potentially migrate.

Screws vary in their diameter and design. Generally, larger-diameter screws with deeper threads and a larger thread pitch are used in cancellous bone, whereas smaller-diameter screws with shallow threads and a narrower pitch are used in cortical bone. Screws may also be cannulated, allowing insertion of the screw over a guide wire.

Many different plates are available for use in fixating fractures. They vary in shape, design, thickness, and composition. The location and nature of the fracture dictates the type of plate used (Figs. 3–4 through 3–18).

Text continued on page 54

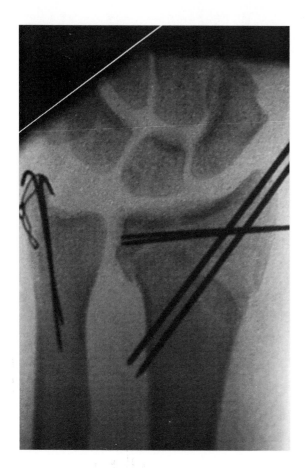

FIGURE 3–4 Smooth Kirschner wires have been used to stabilize this distal radius fracture after closed reduction. Kirschner wires and narrow-gauge malleable wire have also been used to repair an ulnar styloid fracture. This film was obtained from fluoroscopic image that was made during the surgical procedure to confirm the reduction and the wires' positions.

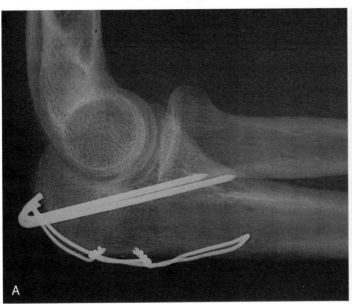
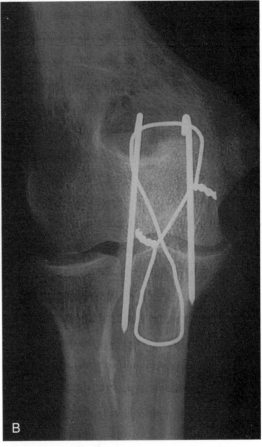

FIGURE 3–5 A: A tension band wire technique has been used to repair this olecranon fracture. The malleable wire has been passed through a drill hole in the ulnar metaphysis and wrapped around the ends of the Kirschner wires. This construct converts the pull of the triceps into a compressive force across the fracture site. Tension band wiring is commonly used for fixation of olecranon and patella fractures, but it requires a stable fracture pattern. Plate fixation may be required in severely comminuted olecranon fractures. **B:** An AP view shows that the malleable wire has been placed in a figure-of-eight fashion around the Kirschner wire. This wire has been tightened by twisting it both medially and laterally.

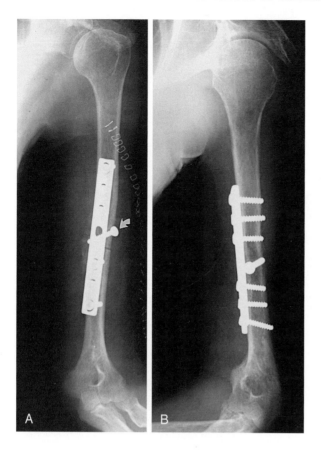

FIGURE 3–6   A: One of the basic tenets of fracture fixation is the achievement of interfragmentary compression. This is commonly managed by using a lag screw. A larger gliding hole is drilled in the near cortex so that the screw threads do not engage the near cortex. The screw threads engage only the far cortex, and as the screw is tightened, compression of the fracture site occurs. This radiograph shows a lag screw (arrow) that transverses the major fracture line. A compression plate is also used because a single lag screw is insufficient fixation to resist the forces of the muscles. Dynamic compression plates are commonly used for long-bone fractures in the upper extremities. These plates have specially designed screw holes that provide slight longitudinal compression of the fracture site as the screws are inserted. The plates vary in their width and thickness and are available in a variety of lengths. The length of plate used is determined by the number of screws necessary on each side of the fracture to achieve adequate stability. It is usual to use a larger plate on the humerus than on the forearm. Screws of a larger diameter are used with the larger plates. If hardware removal is later required, there is a higher risk of refracture through larger screw holes as compared to smaller screw holes. **B:** A lateral view shows the compression plate sitting directly on the cortex. All screw lengths appear to be appropriate. Because the bone is tubular, some screws may appear to be shorter than others and may appear to incompletely penetrate the cortex. A depth gauge is used intraoperatively to select the appropriate screw length.

FIGURE 3–7   A dynamic hip screw is commonly used for the treatment of intertrochanteric hip fractures. It consists of a large compression screw (solid arrow) that is inserted into the femoral neck and head. The compression screw fits into the barrel of the sideplate (open arrow), which is secured to the femoral shaft. The compression screw can slide within the barrel, resulting in compression of the fracture site as the patient ambulates.

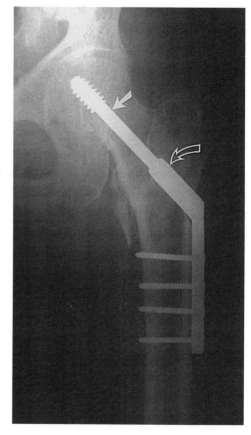

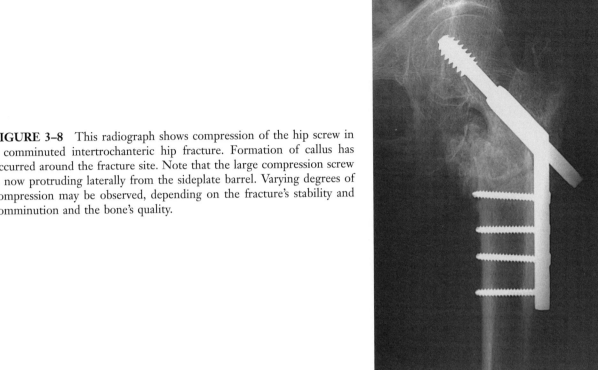

FIGURE 3-8 This radiograph shows compression of the hip screw in a comminuted intertrochanteric hip fracture. Formation of callus has occurred around the fracture site. Note that the large compression screw is now protruding laterally from the sideplate barrel. Varying degrees of compression may be observed, depending on the fracture's stability and comminution and the bone's quality.

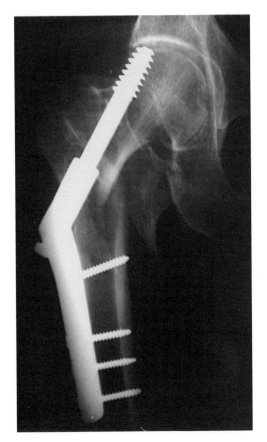

FIGURE 3-9 Occasionally, hip compression screws may "cut out" of the femoral head and begin to erode the acetabulum. This radiograph shows a compression screw that has cut out of the femoral head. A large fragment from a fracture of the lesser trochanteric is seen; it is likely that it compromised the stability of the initial fixation. The patient will require either revision of the fixation or conversion to a hip arthroplasty.

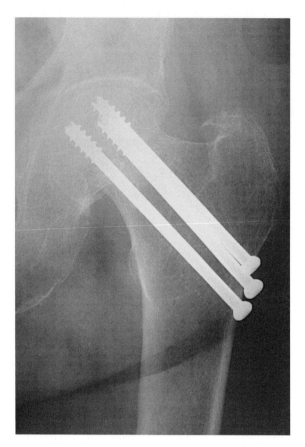

FIGURE 3–10 Cannulated screws have been used to stabilize a minimally displaced femoral neck fracture. These screws may be inserted percutaneously over guide wires that are inserted under fluoroscopic guidance. A fracture table is commonly used to provide traction and maintain fracture reduction during the fixation.

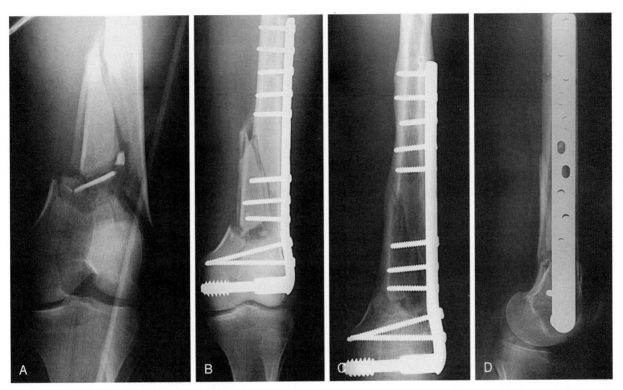

FIGURE 3–11 **A:** A comminuted supracondylar femur fracture. **B:** The fracture has been stabilized with a 95-degree dynamic condylar screw. The intercondylar split was first reduced with smaller lag screws. The large lag screw, which is placed parallel to the joint line, was then inserted. A barrel and sideplate attach to the lag screw and are secured to the femoral shaft. Screws have been inserted into the medial metaphyseal fracture fragment, but no attempt has been made to achieve an anatomic reduction of this fragment. This indirect reduction method minimizes further periosteal stripping so that blood supply to the fracture fragment is maintained. The two basic techniques of fracture reduction are direct reduction and indirect reduction. Direct reduction requires extensive dissection in order to anatomically reduce each fracture fragment. This results in a biomechanically strong construct, but the periosteal stripping can devitalize bone fragments, which delays healing and potentially increases the possibility of infection. In indirect reduction, the articular surface is anatomically reduced and the correct limb alignment is achieved, but no attempt is made to reduce each of the individual fragments. Without periosteal stripping, these comminuted intervening fragments often heal rapidly. In these radiographs, taken 6 weeks postoperatively, early callus formation is seen. **C:** The fracture has healed successfully. Some remodeling of the callus has occurred, as seen on these x-rays taken 10 months postoperatively. **D:** A lateral radiograph shows the correct axial alignment of the implant.

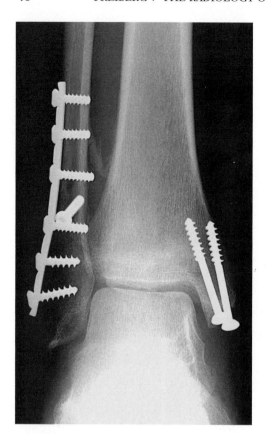

FIGURE 3–12 Displaced bimalleolar ankle fractures are commonly caused by external rotation of a supinated foot. This type of injury is usually treated by open reduction and fixation of the medial malleolus fracture with partially threaded cancellous screws. The fibular fracture is treated with an interfragmentary lag screw and plate fixation using a one-third tubular plate, which is thin and quite malleable. Its purpose is to neutralize the lag screw fixation, not to provide rigid strength.

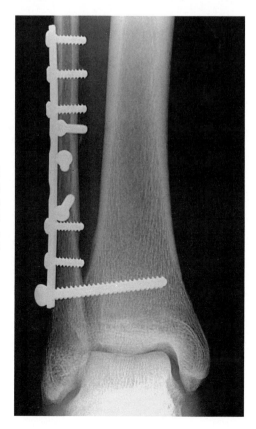

FIGURE 3–13 This bimalleolar ankle fracture resulted from external rotation of a pronated foot. The fibula fracture has occurred well above the ankle joint and caused subsequent disruption of the interosseous membrane between the tibia and fibula. In addition to fixing the fibula and medial malleolus, a temporary fixation screw also secures the fibula to the tibia. This syndesmosis screw is usually removed at 6 to 12 weeks, once the torn interosseous membrane has healed.

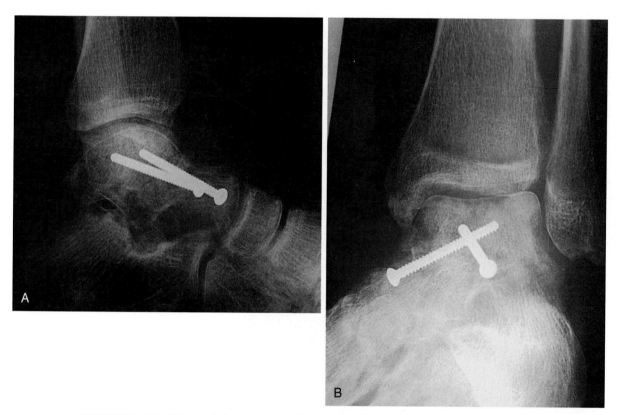

FIGURE 3–14 Talar neck fractures often disrupt the blood supply to the talar body, which runs from the distal to the proximal area. **A:** This lateral radiograph shows anatomic reduction of the talar neck fracture. **B:** Radiolucency, known as a Hawkins' sign, is seen beneath the subchondral surface approximately 3 months postoperatively. This finding indicates successful revascularization of the talar body. During this time, the patient has been nonweightbearing, and disuse osteopenia is present.

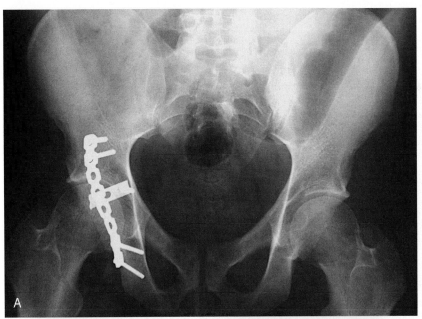

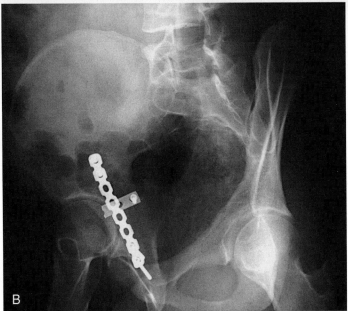

FIGURE 3–15 Reconstruction plates are malleable and are commonly used for the fixation of acetabular and distal humerus fractures. The plates may be shaped to fit irregular surfaces. They do not have the strength of standard compression plates so are rarely used for diaphyseal long-bone fractures, which require stronger implants. **A:** An AP pelvis x-ray shows the reconstruction plate. A portion of a third tubular plate has been fashioned to create a "spring plate." The teeth of this spring plate allow the fixation of small, marginal acetabular fragments. It is used in locations in which screws cannot be safely placed without violating the hip joint. **B:** An iliac oblique Judet view shows the posterior column of the pelvis most clearly. The reconstruction plate is located along the posterior column and is secured above and below the healed posterior wall acetabular fracture.

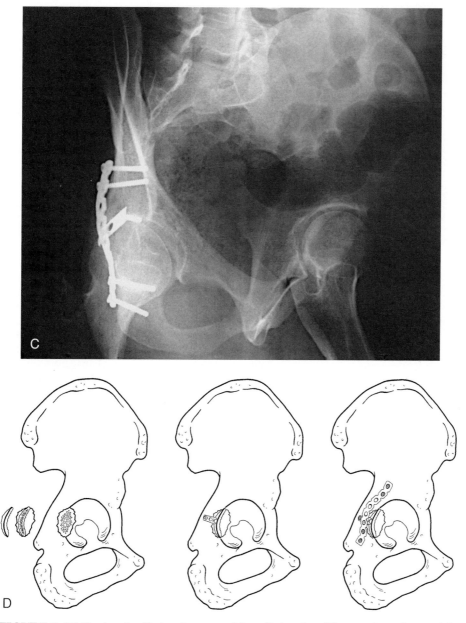

FIGURE 3–15 *Continued.*   **C:** An obturator oblique Judet view. The anterior column of the pelvis is best seen in this view. **D:** A schematic view shows the location of the plate fixation construct on the posterior aspect of the acetabular wall and along the posterior column of the pelvis.

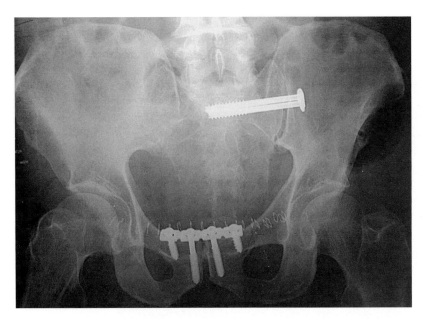

FIGURE 3–16 An open-book pelvic fracture was treated by performing open reduction and internal fixation of the pubic symphysis diastasis. In this case, a large reconstruction plate and 6.5-mm cancellous screws were used. Posteriorly, the widened sacroiliac joint was reduced and fixed with a 7.3-mm cannulated, partially threaded cancellous screw. A washer was used to prevent penetration of the screw head through the cortical bone of the ilium.

FIGURE 3–17 Intraoperative fluoroscopy is used during many surgeries for orthopaedic trauma such as those in which intramedullary nails are employed. Intraoperative plain films may be utilized in many other cases. One of the more common uses of an intraoperative film is to check the overall alignment; an implant may be provisionally fixed and a radiograph obtained to check the alignment before completing the fixation. Films may also be used to check the hardware position and screw lengths. The surrounding regions included in the film should be checked for any injury that was overlooked. This intraoperative film shows a tibial plateau fracture. A distraction device is being used both medially and laterally to assist in the operative procedure. The axial alignment of the joint appears to be normal.

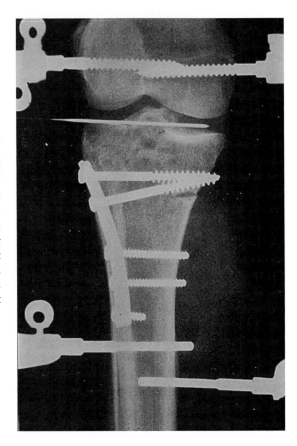

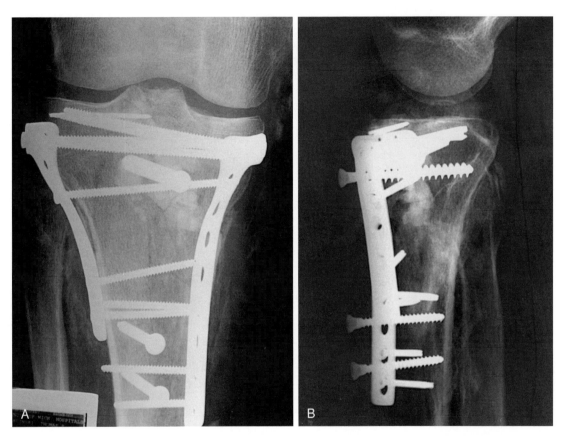

FIGURE 3–18 **A:** An AP view of a severely comminuted bicondylar tibial plateau fracture that has been fixed with both medial and lateral L-shaped buttress plates. Kirschner wires were placed beneath the subchondral surface to piece together small articular fragments. Transverse screws inserted through the holes of the upper plate support the reduced articular surfaces. Pro-Osteon, a coralline hydroxyapatite bone void filler (the square-shaped denser areas in the metaphysis), has been used to fill the metaphyseal defect created by compression of the cancellous bone. Reduction of the articular surface is a critical goal in all periarticular fractures so as to prevent posttraumatic arthritis. Restoration of the anatomic axis is also important. A small degree of varus alignment is present in this case. **B:** A lateral view shows three anterior-to-posterior screws that have been used to secure the separate tibial tubercle fragment.

Intramedullary Fixation

Intramedullary fixation devices are commonly referred to as nails or rods. They are used most commonly for fixation of diaphyseal femoral shaft or tibia fractures. They may also be utilized for humerus and forearm fractures. These devices provide significant benefit to the patient, commonly allowing early weightbearing. Their intramedullary location provides the optimal biomechanical position for resisting torsion and bending.

Early intramedullary fixation devices were solid, without proximal or distal interlocking screws. This limited their use to stable middiaphyseal fractures. Contemporary intramedullary nails allow placement of interlocking screws through holes in the nail. This prevents shortening, angulation, and rotation of the fracture and extends the indications for the use of intramedullary nails to more complex fractures. The screws nearest the insertion site can usually be inserted using an outrigger jig that is attached to the nail insertion device. The screws farthest from the insertion site have to be inserted in a freehand fashion because there is usually too much deformation of the nail to allow the use of an outrigger jig. This freehand insertion is performed using intraoperative fluoroscopy. If the screws fail to engage the nail (if they accidentally fail to pass through the hole), the fracture may shorten, rotate, or angulate.

The insertion of an intramedullary device requires the creation of an entrance site. The tibial entrance site is located proximally, just below the joint line. Femoral nails are most commonly inserted through a proximal entrance site in the piriformis fossa (antegrade) but occasionally may be inserted distally through the intercondylar notch (retrograde). A flexible guide wire is often passed into the intramedullary canal. The intramedullary canal may be enlarged by mechanical reamers to allow insertion of a larger-diameter, and thus stronger, intramedullary nail (Figs. 3–19 through 3–22).

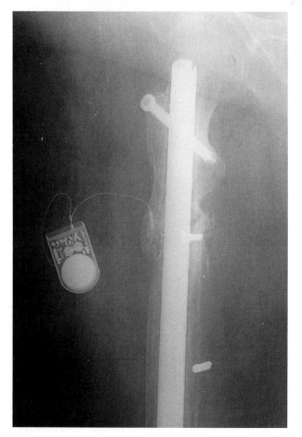

FIGURE 3–19 An implanted electrical stimulator may occasionally be used to provide additional stimulus for growth so as to achieve union in the presence of a nonunion or a spine fusion. This device consists of a battery, which is usually placed subcutaneously, and two wires, the cathode and the anode, which are tunneled through to the desired location. This radiograph shows an implanted electrical stimulator that was inserted for the treatment of a subtrochanteric nonunion. Incidental notation is made of the presence of two broken screw fragments from a failed fixation device.

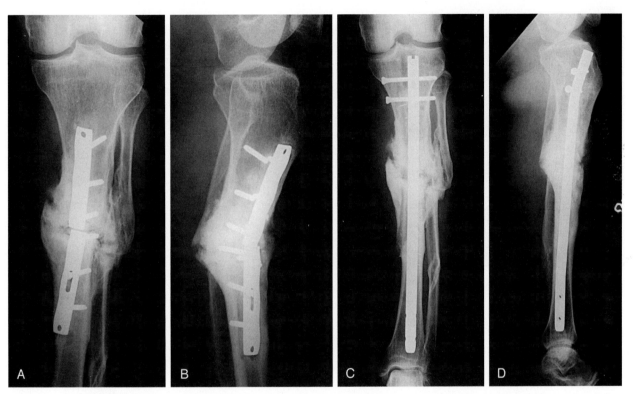

FIGURE 3–20 **A:** This tibial fracture had been treated approximately 30 years earlier with plate fixation; it subsequently developed a nonunion that would be classified as hypertrophic because of the abundant callus present. The plate has suffered a fatigue fracture at the nonunion site. **B:** This lateral view shows a recurvatum deformity at the nonunion site and confirms that several of the screws have broken. After internal fracture fixation, there is a race between fracture healing and implant failure. No implant is strong enough to resist the continuous mechanical demands of weightbearing, and fatigue failure of the implant will occur if the fracture does not heal. Implants usually fail at their weakest point, commonly at a screw hole. Narrow-diameter screws usually are the weakest links and are commonly the first hardware to fail. If there is significant motion at the nonunion site, erosion of the bone may occur, and reactive bone formation may develop around the implant. **C:** This nonunion was treated by removing the broken plate and screws and placing a reamed intramedullary nail. Only the proximal interlocking screws have been placed. Continued compression is achieved at the nonunion site as the patient bears weight. **D:** A lateral view shows correction of the recurvatum deformity.

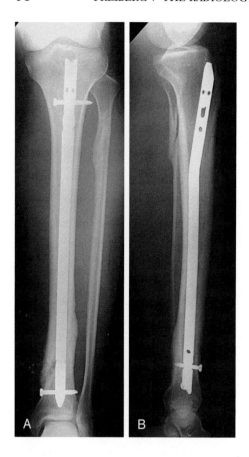

FIGURE 3–21   A: An intramedullary tibial nail has been used to treat this distal spiral tibial fracture. This particular intramedullary nail has several different proximal and distal interlocking options. Because of the very distal location of this fracture, distal interlocking has been performed with one medial-to-lateral screw and one anterior-to-posterior screw. The fracture has achieved a successful union. **B:** A lateral view shows the proximal and distal interlocking holes. A single proximal interlocking screw has been placed in the oval slot; this permits dynamic compression of the fracture site—that is, the interlocking screw can slide within the nail slot as the fracture compresses.

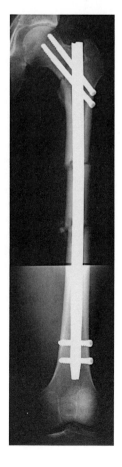

FIGURE 3–22   The patient in this figure has sustained a segmental femoral shaft fracture and an ipsilateral femoral neck fracture. The three fractures have been treated with a special type of intramedullary nail that also allows fixation of fractures around the hip. These nails, referred to as reconstruction nails, allow screws to be placed through the proximal nail and into the femoral neck and head. Reconstruction nails are also indicated in the treatment of subtrochanteric fractures, as additional proximal fixation is often required in these fracture patterns. Reconstruction nails can be used to prophylactically stabilize an impending fracture caused by metastatic disease.

BIBLIOGRAPHY

Browner BD, Jupiter JB, Levine AM, et al. Skeletal Trauma, 2nd ed. Philadelphia: WB Saunders, 1998.

Hansen ST Jr, Swiontkowski MF. Orthopaedic Trauma Protocols. New York: Raven Press, 1993.

Müller MT, Allgöwer M, Schneider R, et al. Manual of Internal Fixation, 3rd ed. Berlin: Springer-Verlag, 1990.

Rockwood CA, Green DP, Bucholz RW, et al., eds. Fractures in Adults, 4th ed. Philadelphia: Lippincott-Raven, 1996.

Wiss DA, ed. Fractures. Philadelphia: Lippincott-Raven, 1998.

4

Sports Medicine: Implants of Knee Ligament Repair and Reconstructive Surgery

JON K. SEKIYA

EDWARD M. WOJTYS

Several bone and soft-tissue fixation techniques have been developed for knee ligament repair, reconstruction, and patellofemoral realignment surgery. A successful outcome of reconstructive surgery of a knee ligament depends on a number of variables. Adequate strength of fixation is essential to prevent failure of the construct. Commonly, the weakest link in reconstructive surgery of a knee ligament is the graft fixation site.[1] As a result, studies have been performed to determine the strongest method of fixation. The technique of using an interference screw with suture fixation of the bone plug in the bone/patellar tendon/bone graft was observed to have the highest mechanical strength and to most closely approximate the normal stiffness of the anterior cruciate ligament (ACL).[1, 2]

In reconstructive surgery of the knees, a factor that is critically linked to the clinical outcome is anatomic tunnel and graft placement. Careful reproduction of ligament anatomy is the goal of reconstructive knee surgery. For instance, the femoral attachment of the ACL originates in the posterior part of the medial surface of the lateral femoral condyle.[3, 4] The attachment is, on average, 15 mm from the "over-the-top" position (the junction between the posterior aspect of the femoral shaft and the most proximal portion of the lateral femoral condyle) and is well posterior in the intercondylar notch.[3] The native ACL attaches to the tibia in a wide area just posterior and lateral to the medial tibial eminence.[3, 4]

The appropriate placement of the center of the femoral tunnel in ACL surgery is debatable, but a good target is the one o'clock to one-thirty position in the left knee and the ten-thirty to eleven o'clock position in the right knee, from the frontal view of the notch. The center of the tibial tunnel should lie in the middle to posterior third of the ACL footprint, or approximately 5 to 7 mm anterior to the posterior cruciate ligament (PCL) at a position one third to one half the distance across the notch, from medial to lateral.[3] Anterior positioning of the graft can lead to impingement of the reconstructed ACL on the femoral notch.[5] In addition, the oblique orientation of the graft must be maintained in order to prevent a vertical ACL reconstruction that usually leads to loss of rotational control. This oblique orientation is dictated by both tibial and femoral graft positioning. At the time of surgery, notchplasty may be performed in order to allow proper visualization of the over-the-top position and minimize impingement of the graft.[3, 5]

Proximally, the PCL is attached to the lateral surface of the medial femoral condyle.[4, 6, 7] Distally, the PCL is attached to an inferior depression behind the intra-articular upper surface of the posterior aspect of the tibia, and it extends approximately 8 mm below the joint line and 3 mm lateral to the midline of the lateral tibial tubercle.[4, 6, 8] The broad PCL may be divided into two parts, the anterolateral and posteromedial bundles.[7]

Anatomic reapproximation of the PCL tibial attachment is difficult in both open and arthroscopic techniques. Proper graft placement at the proximal portion of the tibia is crucial to the prevention of graft failure. Tibial tunnel techniques may place high stress on the tendon/bone interface. Because of its broad origin on the femur, reconstruction of the PCL with a single graft produces only partial PCL function when tested biomechanically. Thus, single-graft reconstructions are unlikely to reproduce normal PCL biomechanics.[7, 9] Reconstruction of both the anterolateral and posteromedial band, with a double bundle graft and two separate femoral attachments, may provide the closest approximation of biomechanical PCL function.

The posterolateral structures of the knee include the lateral collateral ligament (LCL), arcuate ligament, fabellofibular ligament, and popliteus muscle complex.[10, 11] The native LCL is attached proximally in a fanlike shape between the lateral femoral epicondyle and the supracondylar process.[11] The proximal aspect of the LCL is closely associated and connected with the aponeurotic bands of the short and long heads of the biceps femoris muscle. Distally, the medial fibers attach onto the lateral edge of the fibular styloid; the lateral fibers continue distally, blending with the superficial fascia of the lateral compartment of the leg.[10–12]

The arcuate ligament is composed of a medial and a lateral limb that cross over and are firmly adherent to the underlying popliteus complex. The lateral limb attaches distally to the fibular styloid just anterior to the fabellofibular ligament and arches proximally and medially to attach to the posterior joint capsule, just proximal to the popliteal/musculotendinous junction at the level of the superior edge of the posterior horn of the lateral meniscus.[10, 11] The medial limb fans out medially from the fibular styloid and blends proximally with the oblique popliteal ligament from the medial side of the knee.[10, 11]

When the fabellofibular ligament is present, it originates from the lateral edge of the fabella and courses distally and laterally to attach onto the fibular styloid. If no fabella is present, the fabellofibular ligament attaches to the posterior aspect of the supracondylar process of the femur and blends with the anterior fibers of the lateral head of the gastrocnemius tendon.[10, 11]

The popliteus muscle complex consists of the popliteus muscle-tendon unit and the popliteofibular ligament. The popliteofibular ligament arises from the popliteal tendon and inserts into the most posterosuperior aspect of the fibular head.[11, 13] The popliteus muscle originates from the posteromedial surface of the proximal tibia and ascends proximally and laterally, inserting in the popliteal groove of the femur.[10, 11, 13]

The soft tissue on the medial side of the knee can be divided into three layers. The superficial layer consists of the superficial fascia and the sartorius, gracilis, and semitendinosus muscles, known as the pes anserinus. The pes anserinus extends distally to cover the distal attachment of the medial collateral ligament (MCL). The middle layer consists of the superficial MCL, the semimembranosus, and the patellofemoral ligament. The superficial MCL arises from the medial femoral condyle and attaches to the tibia 5 to 7 cm below the joint line, deep to the pes anserinus. The deep layer consists of the joint capsule, the deep MCL, the coronary ligament (meniscotibial ligament), and the posterior oblique fibers, which thicken and blend into the posterior capsule of the knee joint.[14, 15]

The patellar tendon arises mainly from the central fibers of the rectus femoris muscle, with some contributions from the vastus lateralis, and extends distally and anteriorly over the patella. It inserts into the tibial tubercle and blends distally with the fascia of the iliotibial tract on the anterior tibia.[16]

In the radiographic examples, proper graft placement for ligamentous reconstructions are emphasized in light of the previous anatomic descriptions. The first set of radiographs depicts the various origin and insertion sites of key ligamentous structures of the knee that are frequently reconstructed and repaired. They can be used as reference points. These radiographs provide a broad variety of cases that illustrate the many methods used and that display the fixation techniques currently used in knee ligament reconstructive and reparative surgery (Figs. 4–1 through 4–12).

Text continued on page 71

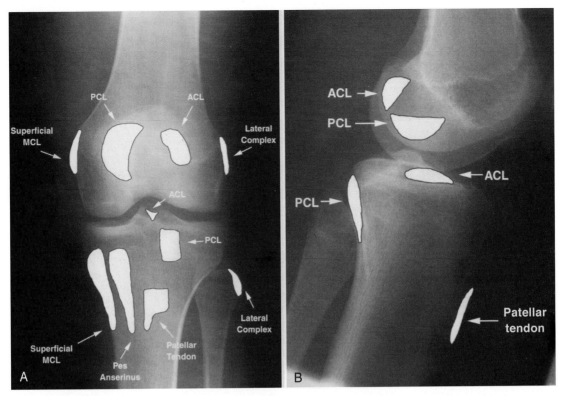

FIGURE 4–1 A and **B:** A normal left knee in a skeletally mature 15-year-old female; physeal scars are visible and growth plates are closed. The origin and insertion sites of knee ligaments that are commonly reconstructed and repaired are labeled. They are to be used as reference points for comparison with the subsequent examples of knee ligament reconstruction and repair.

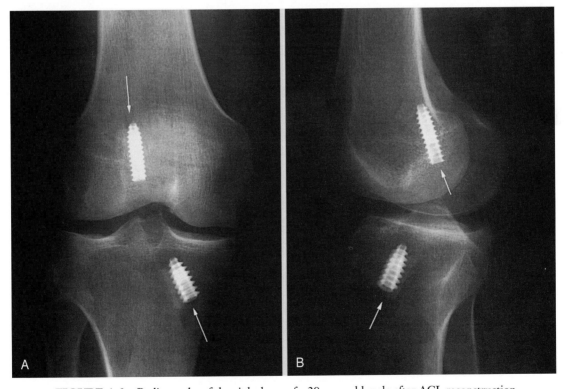

FIGURE 4–2 Radiographs of the right knee of a 29-year-old male after ACL reconstruction with patellar tendon autograft. Interference screws fix the bone/patellar tendon/bone graft both proximally and distally. There is good interference-screw bone-plug alignment without divergence. **A:** The oblique orientation of the graft is to be noted in the posteroanterior (PA) radiograph. **B:** The positioning of the proximal interference screw and femoral bone plug against the posterior cortex of the lateral femoral condyle is seen in the lateral view.

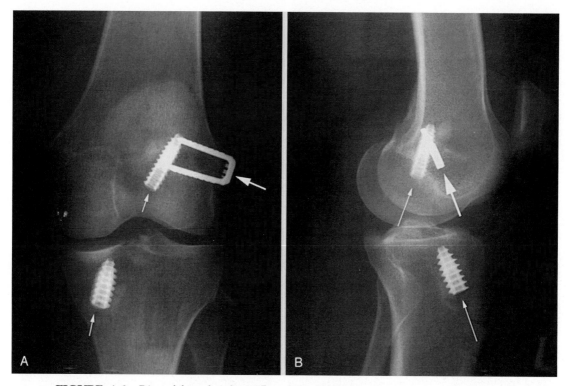

FIGURE 4–3 PA and lateral radiographs of the left knee of a 28-year-old female after ACL reconstruction with patellar tendon autograft and LCL and popliteus complex repair. Interference screws fix the bone/patellar tendon/bone graft both proximally and distally (small arrow). There is slight divergence between the tibial and femoral bone plugs and the interference screw fixation. **A:** The oblique orientation of the graft may be seen in the PA radiograph. **B:** The positioning of the proximal interference screw against the posterior cortex of the lateral femoral condyle may be seen in the lateral view. The LCL and popliteus tendon were advanced and fastened to their femoral attachment with a staple (large arrow).

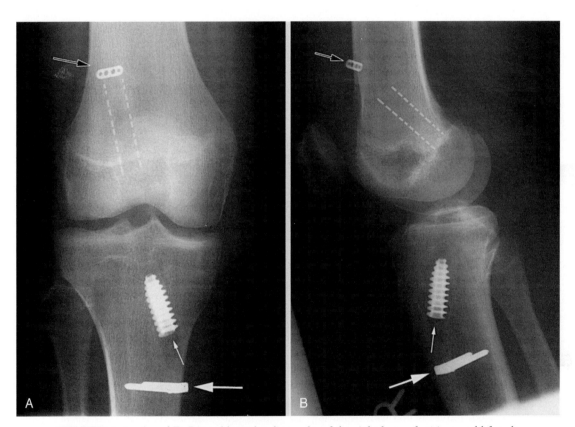

FIGURE 4–4 **A** and **B**: PA and lateral radiographs of the right knee of a 14-year-old female after ACL reconstruction with hamstring autograft. An interference screw (small arrow) and staple (large arrow) stabilize the distal graft. An endobutton (black arrow) is used to fixate the proximal hamstring graft. The femoral tunnel is outlined.

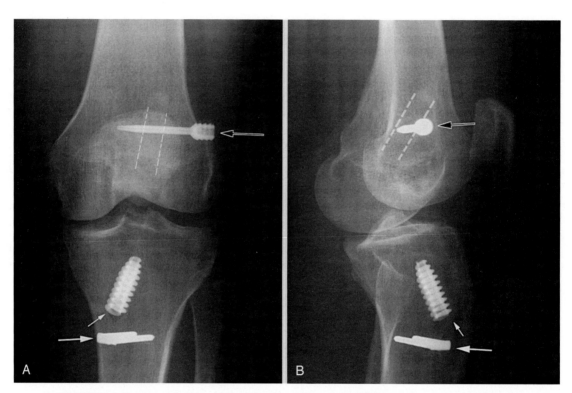

FIGURE 4–5 **A** and **B:** PA and lateral radiographs of the left knee of a 32-year-old female after ACL reconstruction with hamstring autograft. A soft-tissue interference screw (small arrow) and staple (large arrow) stabilize the distal graft. Soft-tissue interference screws have rounded threads that protect the graft. A transfixion pin (black arrow) is used to fixate the proximal hamstring graft. The femoral tunnel is outlined by dotted lines. The position of the femoral tunnel against the posterior cortex of the lateral femoral condyle is to be noted.

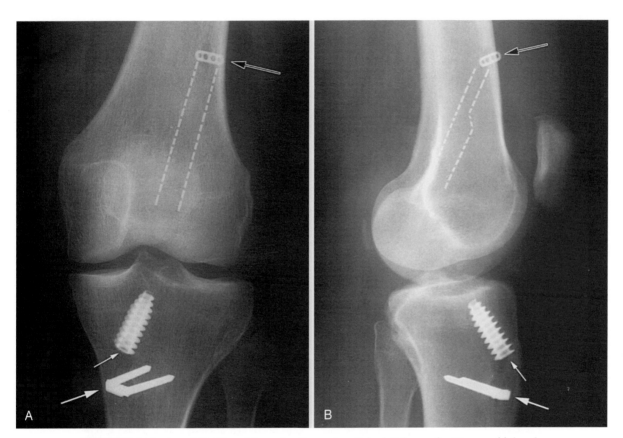

FIGURE 4–6 **A** and **B:** PA and lateral radiographs of the left knee of a 52-year-old female after ACL reconstruction with hamstring autograft. An interference screw (small arrow) and staple (large arrow) stabilize the distal graft. There is slight divergence in the interference-screw/distal-graft engagement position. An endobutton (black arrow) is used to fixate the proximal hamstring graft. The femoral tunnel is outlined.

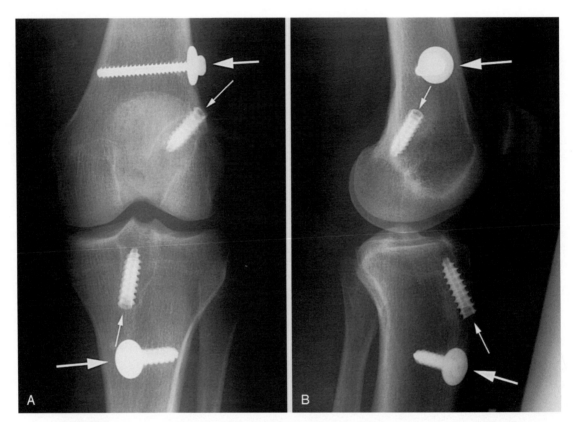

FIGURE 4–7   A and **B:** PA and lateral radiographs of the left knee of a 29-year-old female after ACL reconstruction with patellar tendon allograft. Interference screws (small arrows) fixate the graft through the femoral and tibial tunnels. The tibial interference screw has overpenetrated into the tunnel, partially engaging the tibial bone plug. Cancellous screws and washers (large arrows) are used as posts for sutures, which are threaded through the graft for additional stabilization of the proximal and distal ends.

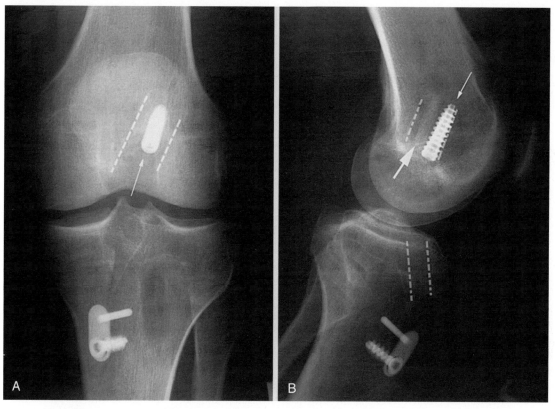

FIGURE 4–8 A and **B:** PA and lateral radiographs of the left knee of a 28-year-old male after ACL reconstruction. The anterior position of the femoral interference screw (small arrow) and bone plug (large arrow) is to be noted. The femoral and tibial tunnels were placed anterior to their anatomic positions (dashed lines) and can contribute to impingement of the graft in the notch, which can lead to loss of terminal extension and early graft failure.

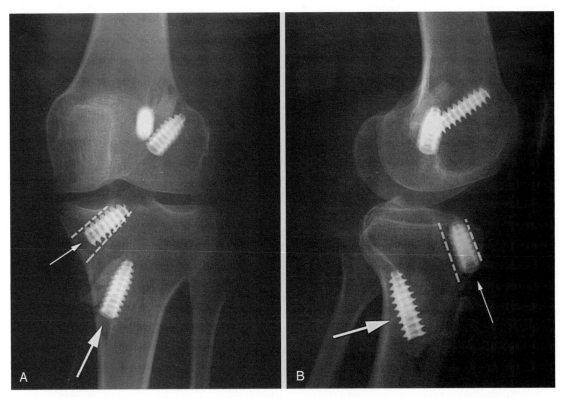

FIGURE 4–9   A and **B:** PA and lateral radiographs of the left knee of a 25-year-old female after revision ACL reconstruction with patellar tendon allograft. Her initial surgery was performed at another institution. Notice the anterior positioning of the tibial tunnel (dashed lines) and interference screw (small arrow). This anterior positioning of the tibial graft can contribute to impingement of the graft on the femoral condyle, which can lead to loss of terminal extension and early graft failure. The new tibial tunnel, interference screw, and graft were placed posterior to the anatomic attachment in order to adequately clear the previous tunnel (large arrow).

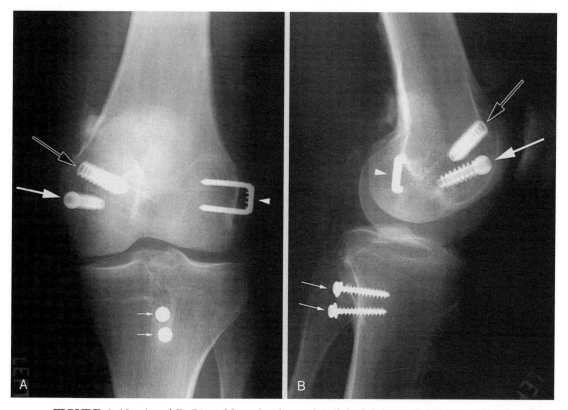

FIGURE 4–10   A and **B:** PA and lateral radiographs of the left knee of a 19-year-old male after PCL reconstruction and MCL and LCL repair required by a knee dislocation sustained in the crash of an all-terrain vehicle. The patient underwent PCL reconstruction with a double-bundle quadriceps tendon graft. Two cancellous screws with washers stabilize the graft to the posterior cortex of the proximal tibia in the area of its anatomic insertion (small arrows). A soft-tissue interference screw (large arrow) stabilizes the anterior femoral graft, and an interference screw (black arrow) stabilizes the posterior graft to the medial femoral condyle. The anterior graft was tightened with the knee near full extension, and the posterior graft was tightened with the knee in 90 degrees of flexion, with the knee reduced in the AP plane. The MCL and medial capsule were repaired with nonabsorbable suture, and the LCL and popliteus complex were advanced and fastened to their femoral attachment with a staple (arrowhead). The staple was placed with the knee in 90 degrees of flexion. In extension, it appears vertical and slightly posterior and inferior.

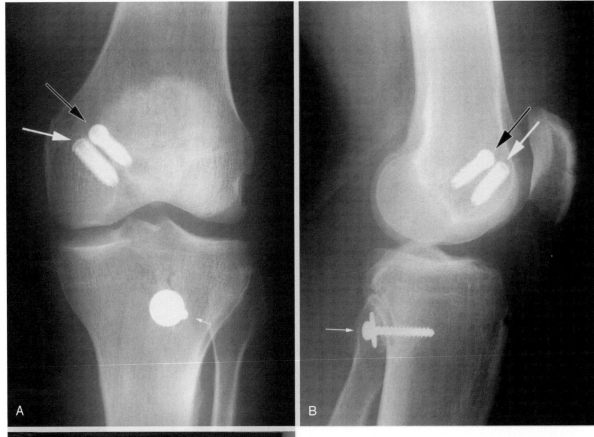

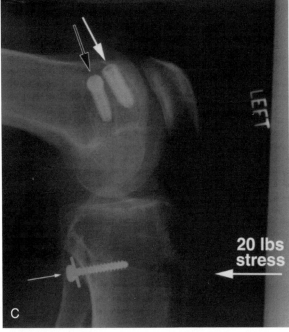

FIGURE 4–11 A, B, and **C:** PA, lateral, and stress-lateral (20 pounds) radiographs of the left knee of a 33-year-old male after PCL reconstruction and MCL repair required by a knee dislocation sustained in an automobile accident. The patient underwent PCL reconstruction and a double-bundle quadriceps tendon graft. A cancellous screw with washer fixates the patella bone plug of the double-bundle quadriceps tendon graft to the posterior cortex of the proximal tibia (small arrow). A soft-tissue interference screw (black arrow) stabilizes the posteromedial bundle, and an interference screw (large arrow) stabilizes the graft of the anterolateral bundle of the quadriceps tendon to the medial femoral condyle. The position of the femoral grafts and how they correlate with the anatomic femoral attachments of the anterolateral and posteromedial bundles are to be noted. The MCL and medial capsule were repaired with nonabsorbable suture.

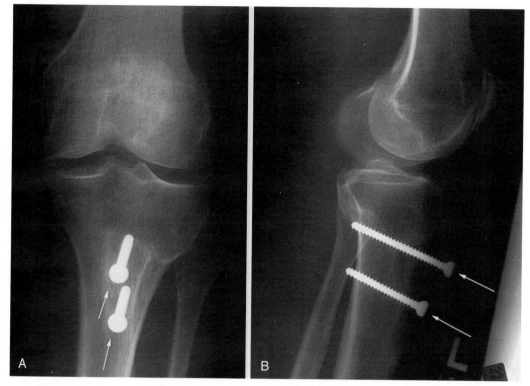

FIGURE 4–12 A and **B:** PA and lateral radiographs of the left knee of a 47-year-old female after anterior medial tibial tubercle transfer, Fulkerson type, for recurrent patellar dislocations.[17] Two 4.5-mm cortical lag screws were used for fixation of the transferred tibial tubercle (arrow). Bicortical purchase of the lag screws is demonstrated, with slight overpenetration of the distal screw. Care must be taken not to overpenetrate the posterior cortex when drilling or tapping or when placing the screws so as to avoid injury to the neurovascular structures that are in close proximity.

REFERENCES

1. Kurosaka M, Yoshiya S, Andrish JT. A biomechanical comparison of different surgical techniques of graft fixation in anterior cruciate ligament reconstruction. Am J Sports Med 1987;15:225–229.
2. Steiner ME, Hecker AT, Brown CH, et al. Anterior cruciate ligament graft fixation: comparison of hamstring and patellar tendon grafts. Am J Sports Med 1994;22:240–246.
3. Dodds JA, Arnoczky SP. Anatomy of the anterior cruciate ligament: a blueprint for repair and reconstruction. Arthroscopy 1994;10:132–139.
4. Girgis FG, Marshall JL, Al Monajem ARS. The cruciate ligaments of the knee joint: anatomical, functional and experimental analysis. Clin Orthop 1975;106:216–231.
5. Howell SM, Clark JA, Farley TE. A rationale for predicting anterior cruciate graft impingement by the intercondylar roof: a magnetic resonance imaging study. Am J Sports Med 1991;19:276–282.
6. Covey DC, Sapega AA. Anatomy and function of the posterior cruciate ligament. Clin Sports Med 1994;13:509–518.
7. Miller MD, Harner CD. The anatomic and surgical considerations for posterior cruciate ligament reconstruction. Instr Course Lect 1995;44:431–440.
8. Racanelli JA, Drez D. Posterior cruciate ligament tibial attachment anatomy and radiographic landmarks for tibial tunnel placement in PCL reconstruction. Arthroscopy 1994;10:546–549.
9. Covey DC, Sapega AA, Sherman GM. Testing for isometry during reconstruction of the posterior cruciate ligament: anatomic and biomechanical considerations. Am J Sports Med 1996;24:740–746.
10. Seebacher JR, Inglis AE, Marshall JL, et al. The structure of the posterolateral aspect of the knee. J Bone Joint Surg 1982;64A:536–541.
11. Terry GC, LaPrade RF. The posterolateral aspect of the knee: anatomy and surgical approach. Am J Sports Med 1996;24:732–739.
12. Kaplan EB. Some aspects of functional anatomy of the human knee joint. Clin Orthop 1962;23:18–29.
13. Maynard MJ, Deng X, Wickiewicz TL, et al. The popliteofibular ligament: rediscovery of a key element in posterolateral stability. Am J Sports Med 1996;24:311–316.

14. Warren LF, Marshall JL. The supporting structures and layers on the medial side of the knee: an anatomical analysis. J Bone Joint Surg 1979;61A:56–62.
15. Warren LF, Marshall JL, Girgis F. The prime static stabilizer of the medial side of the knee. J Bone Joint Surg 1974;56A:665–674.
16. Reider B, Marshall JL, Koslin B, et al. The anterior aspect of the knee joint: an anatomical study. J Bone Joint Surg 1981;63A:351–356.
17. Fulkerson JP, Becker GJ, Meaney JA, et al. Anteromedial tibial tubercle transfer without bone graft. Am J Sports Med 1990;18:490–496.

5

The Shoulder

JOHN E. KUHN

JAMES E. CARPENTER

Shoulder Arthroplasty

A variety of options are available to an orthopaedic surgeon when performing shoulder arthroplasty. In general, a shoulder arthroplasty consists of a humeral-side replacement and a glenoid-side replacement. When a humeral replacement is performed without replacing the glenoid, it is known as a hemiarthroplasty of the shoulder (Fig. 5–1). Hemiarthroplasty typically is used in the presence of a normal glenoid—that is, when treating a fracture of the humeral head or when the rotator cuff is severely damaged such as occurs in a case of rotator cuff tear arthropathy. When the humerus and glenoid are replaced concurrently, it is known as a total shoulder arthroplasty (Fig. 5–2).

HUMERAL COMPONENTS

A number of humeral components have been developed; most consist of a humeral stem and a modular humeral head. The humeral stem may be inserted using interference fit, in which case no polymethylmethacrylate cement would be used (see Fig. 5–1). On the other hand, many components and most arthroplasties inserted to treat humeral head fractures are cemented in place (Fig. 5–3). Humeral head resurfacing implants exist and are used in Europe but are not currently approved for use in the United States.

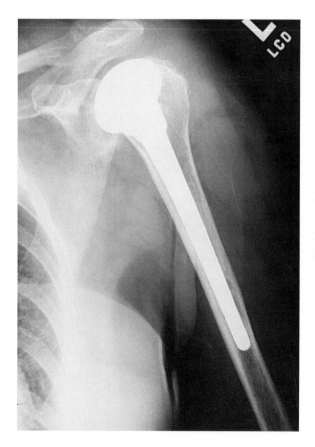

FIGURE 5–1 Hemiarthroplasty of the glenohumeral joint using an interference-fit humeral stem. In this patient, the surgeon elected to replace only the humeral head, and a humeral prosthesis was secured in the humerus by interference fit; no cement was used.

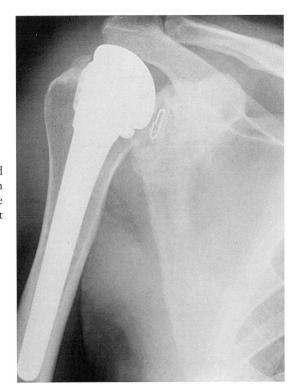

FIGURE 5–2 A total shoulder arthroplasty with a keeled glenoid component. The glenoid can be seen by noting the wire loop in the keel of the glenoid. The glenoid has been cemented into the scapula; the humeral component is an interference fit and does not require cement.

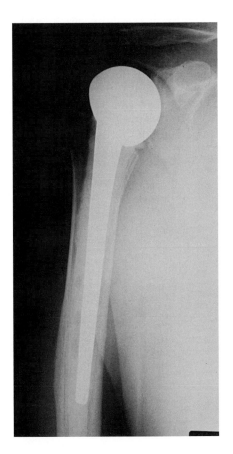

FIGURE 5–3 Cemented humeral stem. Notice the small lucencies next to the component. They probably represent blood that collected during cementing, not loosening of the component.

GLENOID COMPONENTS

Whether to use a glenoid component is left to the surgeon's discretion. In general, glenoid replacement is not performed when a patient requires shoulder arthroplasty because of fracture. Glenoids come in a variety of types, including a metal-backed type that may be secured by screws that are inserted into the glenoid bone stock. Polyethylene glenoids are typically cemented into place. There are two general types: keeled glenoids (Figs. 5–4 through 5–6) and pegged glenoids. It is common for lucencies to appear around the cement mantle; they may be a sign that the glenoid is loosening (see Fig. 5–6).

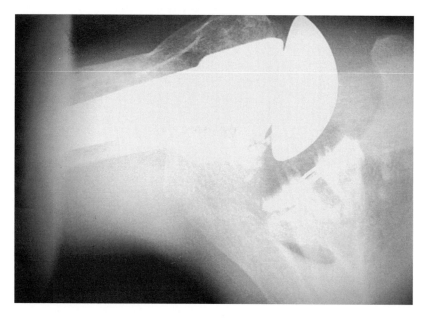

FIGURE 5–4 Axillary view of a total shoulder arthroplasty. The glenoid keel is easily identified by the indwelling wire loop. The glenoid component is cemented in place. Some lucency around the glenoid keel may be present and does not necessarily indicate loosening. Progressive lucencies do indicate loosening (see Fig. 5–6).

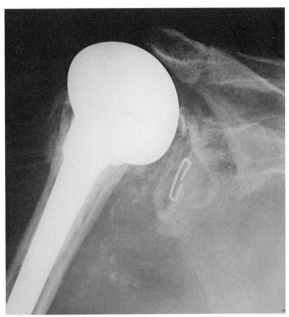

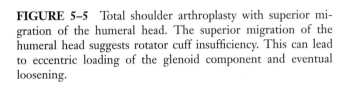
FIGURE 5–5 Total shoulder arthroplasty with superior migration of the humeral head. The superior migration of the humeral head suggests rotator cuff insufficiency. This can lead to eccentric loading of the glenoid component and eventual loosening.

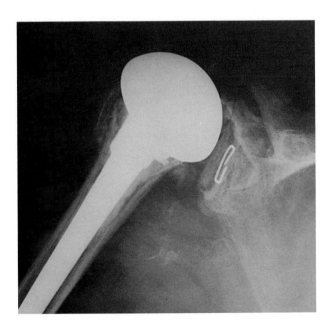

FIGURE 5–6 Total shoulder arthroplasty with superior migration of the humeral head and lucency developing around glenoid. This is the same patient shown in Fig. 5–5. The lucency around the glenoid cement has progressed, suggesting that the glenoid may be loose.

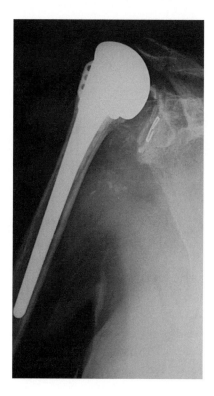

FIGURE 5–7   Severe superior humeral head migration indicating incompetency of the rotator cuff. Migration causes uneven loading on the glenoid component and is commonly associated with lucencies around the cement on the glenoid.

RECOGNIZING COMPLICATIONS IN SHOULDER ARTHROPLASTY

Radiographs may reveal a variety of complications after shoulder arthroplasty. They can include superior migration of the humeral head, which suggests rotator cuff deficiency (Fig. 5–7) and can lead to uneven wear of the glenoid and subsequent loosening; instability of the shoulder arthroplasty (Fig. 5–8); and dislocation of the glenoid component (Fig. 5–9). Intraoperative fractures of the humerus can sometimes be seen (Fig. 5–10). Radiolucent lines around the glenoid keel (see Fig. 5–6) or the humeral shaft may indicate gradual loosening of the arthroplasty; however, the presence of these lines does not correlate with symptoms and may not progress with time.

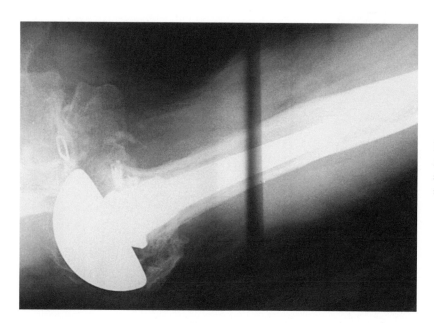

FIGURE 5–8   Axillary view of a posterior dislocation of the humeral prosthesis in a patient with total shoulder arthroplasty.

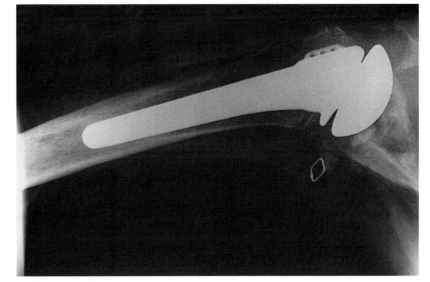

FIGURE 5–9 Axillary view of a total shoulder arthroplasty with dislocation of the glenoid component. The prosthetic glenoid component is marked by the wire loop, which is no longer located in the glenoid bone stock.

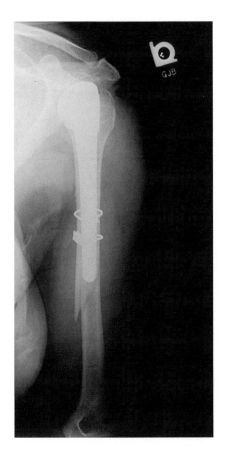

FIGURE 5–10 Shoulder arthroplasty complicated by a spiral fracture of the humerus. In this shoulder, a spiral fracture of the humerus developed during implantation of the humeral component. The fracture was fixed with cerclage wires. An alternative method of treatment is to exchange the humeral component for one with a long intramedullary stem.

Fracture Fixation

FRACTURES OF THE HUMERAL HEAD

A number of techniques are available for the reconstruction of displaced fractures of the humeral head: closed reduction and percutaneous pinning (Fig. 5–11); cerclage wires (Fig. 5–12); and internal fixation using intramedullary nails (Fig. 5–13A and B). Fractures of the lesser tuberosity are typically reduced and held with a single screw (Fig. 5–14A and B). Surgical neck fractures are fixed by means of intramedullary fixation (see Fig. 5–13A and B) or blade plates (Fig. 5–15A and B). For fractures at the anatomic neck with displacement of the humeral head, humeral head hemiarthroplasty is commonly used, as the risk for avascular necrosis of the humeral head is high (Fig. 5–16A and B).

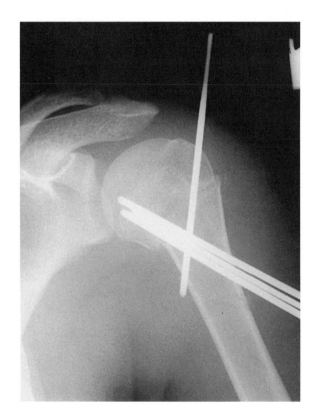

FIGURE 5–11 Fracture of the surgical neck of the humerus held with percutaneous pins. These fractures are typically reduced under fluoroscopy and held with pins, which are placed percutaneously and removed after a number of weeks.

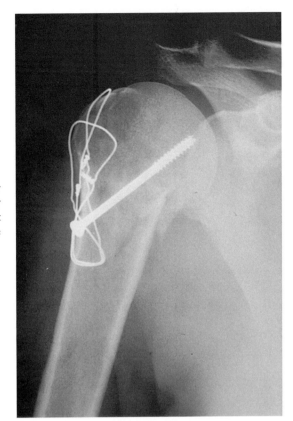

FIGURE 5–12 Tension band wires and a single screw fixation for fracture of the proximal humerus. Tension band wiring is typically reserved for fractures of the tuberosities or surgical neck and is not used for fracture patterns that include the anatomic neck of the proximal humerus.

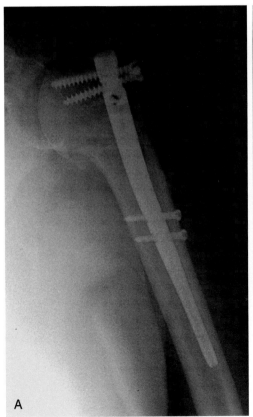

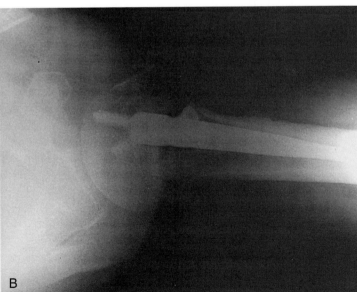

FIGURE 5–13 Intramedullary nail fixation of a fracture of the surgical neck of the humerus. This particular nail is designed to secure fractures of the tuberosities with screws. **A:** Anteroposterior view. **B:** Axillary view.

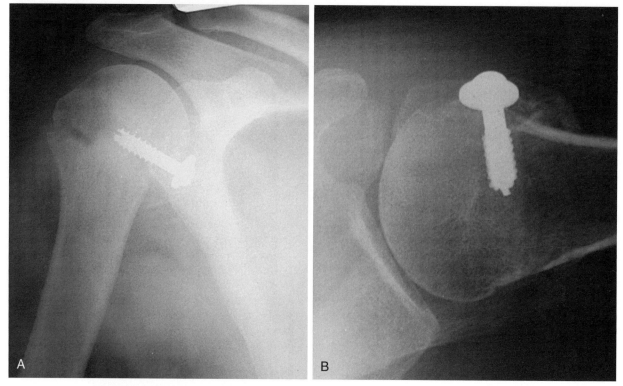

FIGURE 5–14   Single screw fixation of a fracture of the lesser tuberosity of the humerus.
A: Anteroposterior view. **B:** Axillary view.

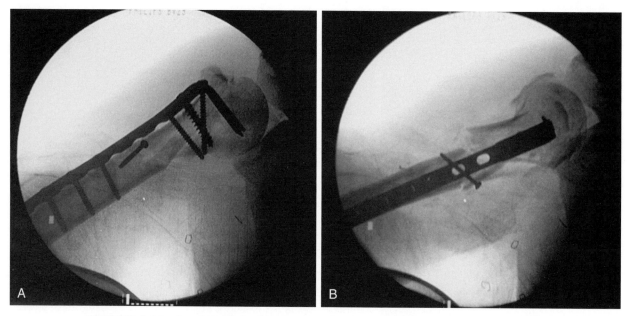

FIGURE 5–15   A and **B:** Blade plate fixation of a comminuted proximal humerus fracture.
This fracture pattern was held with a blade plate, as the extensive comminution made other
fixation methods difficult to perform.

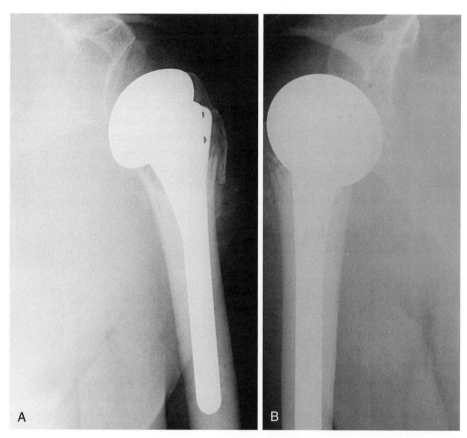

FIGURE 5–16 **A** and **B:** Arthroplasty as treatment of a proximal humerus fracture. Fractures that involve the anatomic neck of the humerus are likely to lead to avascular necrosis of the humeral head if reduced and fixed, so arthroplasty is recommended as the initial treatment. Typically, these fractures include those of the tuberosities, which are sutured to the humeral shaft over the implant; a bone graft from the humeral head may be performed at the same time.

FRACTURES OF THE HUMERAL SHAFT

Fractures of the humeral shaft may be treated by using plating (Fig. 5–17A and B) or intramedullary nails (Fig. 5–18).

Soft-tissue Repairs

IMPLANTS FOR SOFT-TISSUE FIXATION

The musculoskeletal soft tissues play a central role in the function of the shoulder joint. High loads are placed on these soft tissues as a result of the relative lack of joint stability provided by the bony anatomy and the long lever created when forceful activities, such as throwing, are performed at the level of the hand. This explains, in part, why the majority of injuries and sources of disability in the shoulder arise in the soft tissues. Rotator cuff injuries and dislocations are the most common injuries. Their treatment commonly includes repair or reconstruction of the tendons or ligaments. To perform these repairs, attachment of the soft tissue to bone is generally required. In the past, attachment was most commonly achieved by means of direct suturing to a prepared bone surface through osseous tunnels. These techniques are successful, but they are difficult and time consuming. They also require generous surgical exposure of the attachment site.

Bone Staples

Implantable devices to improve the fixation of soft tissue to bone have historically been used less often in the shoulder than in other areas; however, bone staples have

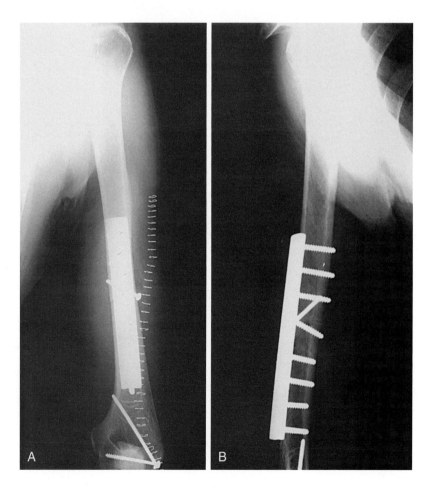

FIGURE 5–17 Plate fixation of a humeral shaft fracture. **A:** Anteroposterior view. **B:** Lateral view.

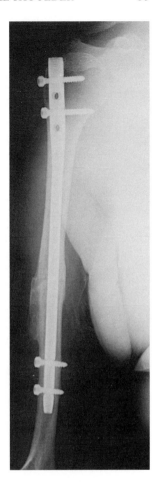

FIGURE 5–18 Intramedullary fixation of humeral shaft fractures. Most intramedullary nails include interlocking screws proximally and distally.

been used when location and size permit. They include subscapularis advancement such as the Magnuson-Stack and modified combined repairs that are used for recurrent dislocations (Fig. 5–19) as well as for some rotator cuff tears. However, the use of such hardware for rotator cuff reattachment can cause mechanical impingement on the acromion process.

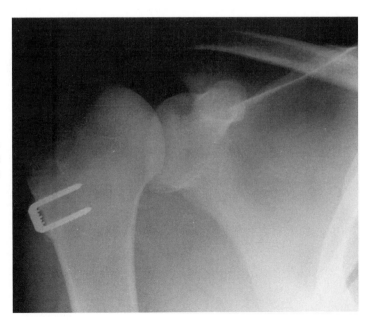

FIGURE 5–19 Use of a staple for soft-tissue fixation. This serrated staple was used to attach the subscapularis tendon to the humerus. Note the small teeth designed to hold the soft tissue.

Bone Screws

Bone screws have also been used to attach soft tissue to bone. Typically, some sort of washer device is used with the screw to provide better fixation to the soft tissue. The washer can be flat and smooth or can have prongs to grip the tissues (Fig. 5–20A and B). Although these screws provide good fixation to bone, the fixation to the soft tissue is usually not ideal. Other techniques that employ screw fixation transfer a portion of bone with the soft tissue still attached (Fig. 5–21), so the fixation occurs between bone and bone, which is a stronger bond than fixation that occurs between soft tissue and bone.

Suture Anchors

In the mid 1980s, devices known as suture anchors were introduced to the market. They are implantable devices designed to rigidly attach a surgical suture to a bone. Approximately 2 to 5 mm in diameter and 3 to 10 mm in length, they are placed directly into the bone or into a predrilled hole, and the attached suture is then used to connect the soft tissues to the bone. It is significantly easier to place suture anchors than it is to create transosseous tunnels: time is saved and limited exposure

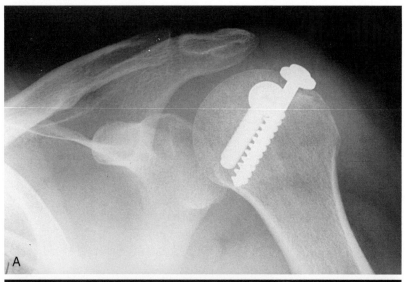

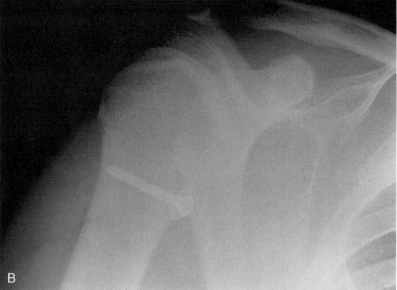

FIGURE 5–20 Use of screws and washers for soft-tissue fixation. Bone screws with washers can provide strong fixation of soft tissues. **A:** Smooth washers increase the area of compression, as in this supraspinatus avulsion with a small amount of bone. **B:** Washers with teeth provide improved holding of the soft tissues. In this example, the washer is mostly radiolucent plastic and has a metal ring for strength.

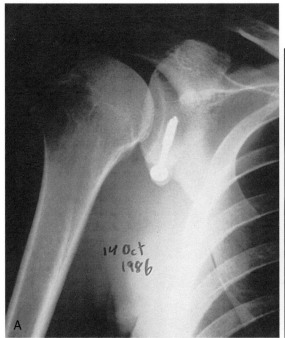 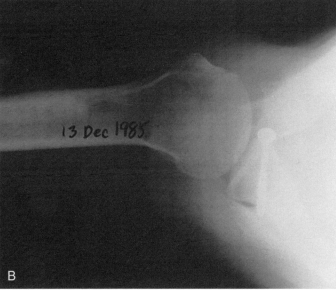

FIGURE 5–21 **A** and **B:** Soft-tissue transfer with bone. Soft-tissue structures can be transferred from one bony attachment to another by transferring a small portion of the bone with the tendon. In this case, because of recurrent dislocations, the conjoined tendon (the coracobrachialis and the short head of the biceps) is transferred to the glenoid rim (the Bristow procedure) with a portion of the coracoid process.

is necessary. Indeed, suture anchors can allow repairs to be performed arthroscopically, thus requiring minimal exposure.

Suture anchors were first introduced by Mitek (Mitek Products, Westwood, MA). They consisted of a metallic body with an eyelet for suture attachment and flexible side arms made of Nitinol, a nickel-titanium alloy (Fig. 5–22). The arms deflect upon insertion and then spring out in the softer cancellous bone, thus preventing removal. With the success of these devices, a large number of additional devices were developed and made available for use. Although the indications are the same, the designs vary widely; expanding flanges and screw threads are the most common designs (Fig. 5–23). An anchor with screw threads on the body has the

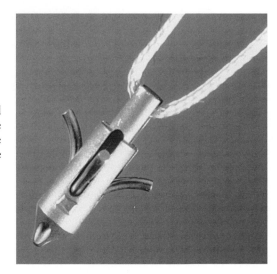

FIGURE 5–22 Suture anchor. This device is known as the G4 and was manufactured by Mitek. It has flexible arms that deflect while being inserted, then spread to prevent pullout from bone. The attached suture can then be used to securely fix soft tissues to the bone surface without the necessity of creating transosseous tunnels.

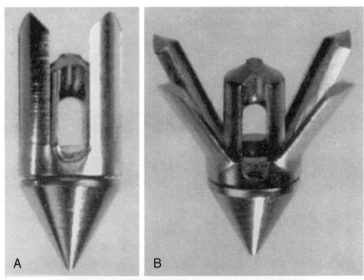

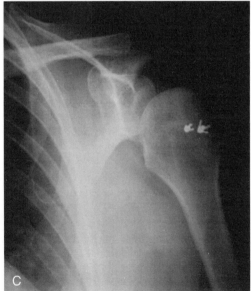

FIGURE 5–23 Expanding suture anchor. **A:** Before deployment. **B:** After deployment. The device is placed into a drilled hole and then expanded, which fixes it within the bone. **C:** An expanding device has been used in the greater tuberosity for rotator cuff attachment.

advantage of being removable if that becomes necessary. Each device has a different appearance on a radiograph, but their placement and function remain the same.

Typical applications for these devices are the attachment of the rotator cuff to the greater tuberosity (Fig. 5–24); the shoulder labrum and capsule to the glenoid rim; and the rotator cuff to the humerus. Suture anchors may be used in other locations in the vicinity of the shoulder in unusual circumstances. Reattachment of the labrum and capsule to the glenoid rim is performed in the case of a traumatic detachment of the labrum (Fig. 5–25). Anterior dislocation is the most common mechanism for such pathology; it results in an anteroinferior detachment commonly known as a Bankart or Perthes lesion. Such a lesion is repaired at the anteroinferior rim of the glenoid. Other labral detachments can occur such as, for example, a superior labrum anteroposterior lesion, in which the tissue disruption is in a more superior location, at the point of attachment of the long head of the biceps tendon to the superior glenoid tubercle. The repair of such an injury, therefore, is performed in a location superior to that of a Bankart lesion (Fig. 5–26).

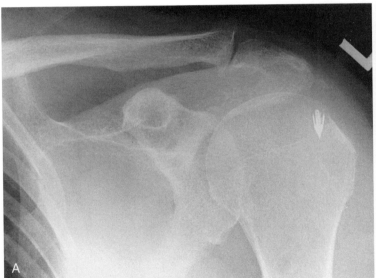
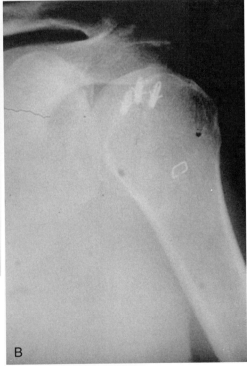

FIGURE 5–24 A and B: Rotator cuff repair with suture anchors. These anchors were placed into the greater tuberosity for reattachment of the supraspinatus. Such devices allow repairs to be completed with less surgical exposure and morbidity than occur when transosseous tunnels must be created.

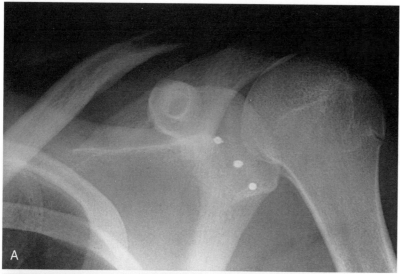

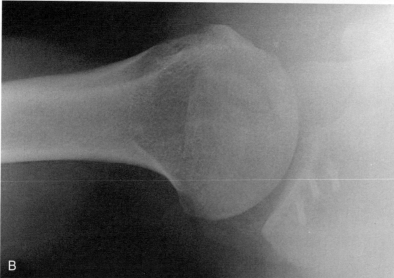

FIGURE 5–25 Bankart lesion repair. Suture anchors are used routinely for repair of the detached glenoid labrum and capsule that are seen with the recurrent dislocations commonly known as Bankart or Perthes lesions. **A:** An anteroposterior view demonstrates insertion along the glenoid rim in the inferior portion of the glenoid, where the detachment typically occurs. **B:** An axillary view demonstrates anterior placement.

FIGURE 5–26 Repair of the superior labrum. Tears of the superior labrum can be repaired by using suture anchors. In this case, screw-in anchors were used. Note the placement in the superior glenoid compared to the location of the Bankart lesion in the anteroinferior location.

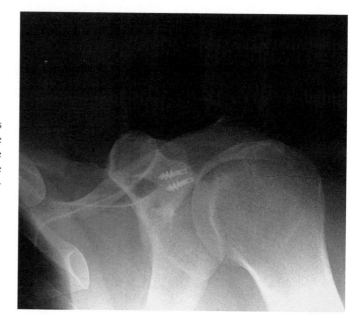

Radiographically, suture anchors should be seen to rest entirely within the bone. When seen outside of the bone in any plane of view, it means the anchor is not fully within bony tissue (Fig. 5–27) and may have become dislodged from the locus of its initial placement or may have been placed outside of the bone at the time of insertion. Generally, an anchor that lies outside of the bone does not cause a problem (see Fig. 5–27A), but if the device becomes positioned in the intra-articular space, injury to the joint surfaces may occur (see Fig. 27B and C). Early recognition and removal of an intra-articular foreign body can help to minimize joint damage. If an anchor is suspected of being in the joint space or other inappropriate place, the area can be further evaluated by performing a computed tomography or fluoroscopy scan (Fig. 5–28).

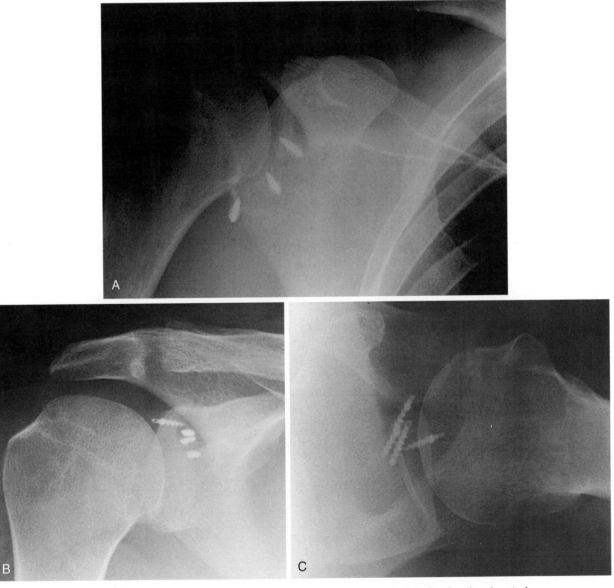

FIGURE 5–27 Anchors outside the bone. Suture anchors are designed to be placed entirely within the bone. **A:** In some locations extraosseus placement causes no problems. **B** and **C:** In other cases, such as in intra-articular placement and when migration has occurred, pain can result. In this case, articular cartilage injury requires further treatment.

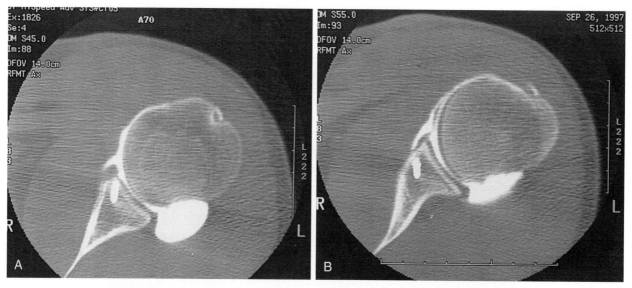

FIGURE 5–28   Computed tomography scan of a suture anchor. Computed tomography can be used to more precisely locate a suture anchor. **A:** For repair of instability, the anchor should be placed at the glenoid rim. **B:** The anchor should *not* be placed down along the neck as shown here.

Acromioclavicular Joint Repairs

Injuries to the acromioclavicular (AC) joint are most commonly ligamentous disruptions of the AC capsule, with or without coracoclavicular ligament tears. Isolated AC capsule injury is known as a grade I sprain or separation. It is universally treated nonsurgically. More severe injuries—grades II through VI—involve more significant displacement and ligament tearing. Although the majority of these injuries are also treated nonsurgically, certain cases are repaired surgically. Techniques are varied and include direct joint transfixion using pins (Fig. 5–29) and coracoclavicular fixation using screws or grafts. As a result of the movement at the AC joint, rigid fixation often leads to fatigue failure of metallic implants if they are not removed once soft-tissue healing is complete (Fig. 5–30). Because of this problem, the most popular techniques currently employ grafts between the clavicle and the coracoid process. The coracoid process, with the attached conjoined tendon, can be transferred to the clavicle and secured with a screw (Fig. 5–31). Both absorbable and nonabsorbable

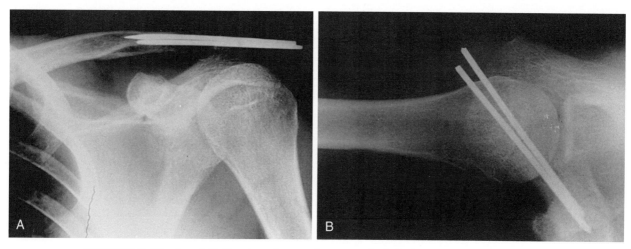

FIGURE 5–29   **A** and **B:** Fixation of a complete acromioclavicular separation. In this case, a posteriorly displaced AC joint separation was reduced and stabilized with threaded pins.

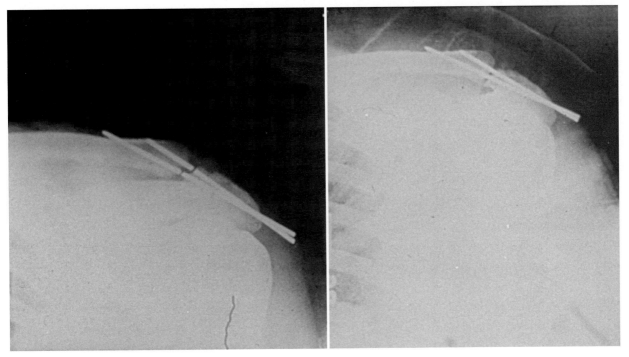

FIGURE 5–30 Failure of pins at the acromioclavicular joint. As a result of joint motion, pins placed across the AC or sternoclavicular joint commonly fail if not removed soon enough. Pin migration into the chest has been seen in some cases.

FIGURE 5–31 Coracoid transfer because of acromioclavicular separation. In this case, the tip of the coracoid process, along with the attached conjoined tendon, is transferred to the clavicle and secured with a screw to stabilize the clavicle.

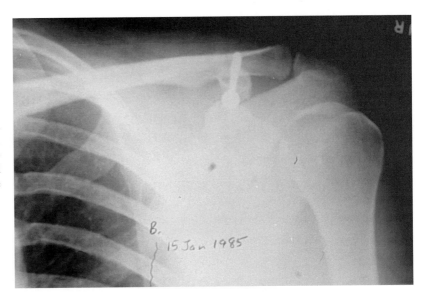

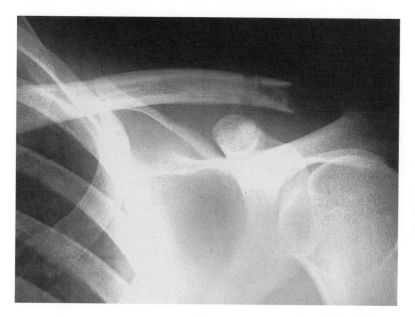

FIGURE 5–32   Graft fixation of acromio-clavicular separation. Radiolucent grafts are commonly used to stabilize the clavicle and the coracoid process. Synthetic or biologic grafts can be used. The only radiographic clue to the graft is the hole created in the distal clavicle for placement of the graft. Often, a distal clavicle resection, with or without the transfer of the coracoclavicular ligament, is also performed.

prosthetic materials as well as biologic grafts (such as the palmaris longus, gracilis, and semitendinosus) have been recommended. In these cases the graft material is radiolucent, so the only radiographic indication of the presence of such a graft is the hole that has been drilled in the clavicle for placement of the graft (Fig. 5–32).

6

Radiology of Total Hip Replacement

ANDREW A. FREIBERG

GREGORY J. GOLLADAY

BRIAN R. HALLSTROM

Total hip arthroplasty is one of the most common and successful orthopaedic surgical procedures currently performed. Total hip implants are assessed on the initial postoperative film and at periodic intervals thereafter. Routine radiographic evaluation of hip replacement is useful to identify signs of wear, loosening, and infection. It is of paramount importance that the evaluator be able to differentiate the normal changes of remodeling from those associated with wear or loosening. The discrimination between normal long-term radiographic changes and implant failure can be complex, as some of the distinctive features of each can overlap.

The femoral component is evaluated for type, position (neutral, varus, valgus), quality of collar-calcar contact, centralization, and the presence of osteolysis. A femoral component is considered to be in varus alignment if the proximal end of the stem is closer to the acetabular implant (tipped away from the greater trochanter) (Diagram A-1). A stem in valgus alignment has its proximal end angled laterally toward the greater trochanter (Diagram A-2). Neutral alignment implies no varus or valgus position, and the proximal and distal portions of the implant are centrally placed (Diagram A-3). The femoral stem should be in neutral position on the anteroposterior (AP) view and should be anteverted approximately 15 to 20 degrees. A symmetric cement mantle should be seen in the presence of cemented components. Cementless components ideally have both proximal and diaphyseal fit and fill. When new radiographs are compared to previous ones, any change in implant position should be noted.

The quality of the cement technique is graded from A to D on the postoperative film according to a modified system developed by Barrack and colleagues.[1] Grade A is a complete white-out of cement such that the cement and cortex are indistinguishable. Grade B indicates near white-out, but cement and cortex are distinct in some areas. This finding results from incomplete filling of the canal. Grade C1 means there are radiolucencies in at least 50% of the cement/bone interface or there are cement bubbles or voids. Grade C2 indicates the presence of a cement mantle less than 1 mm thick in any view. Grade D means major voids exist in the cement mantle. Prostheses with Grades C2 and D are more prone to aseptic loosening than those having Grades A, B, or C1.

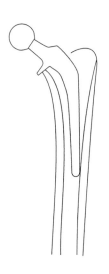
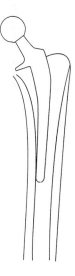
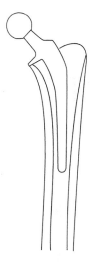

DIAGRAM A–1   DIAGRAM A–2   DIAGRAM A–3

The most common long-term radiographic change in a normal cemented femoral component is the formation of a neocortex between the cement mantle and the inner cortex. This often discontinuous radiodense line can be misidentified as loosening. Resorption of bone, particularly in the calcar region, is common and does not represent a pathologic process. Rather, the bone adjacent to femoral stems is subject to reduced loads and remodels accordingly. This phenomenon is called *stress shielding*. Conversely, substantial normal changes around an acetabular component are rare. New periacetabular radiolucency usually indicates loosening or is a manifestation of the inward migration of polyethylene wear-debris. Osteolysis is the focal resorption of bone through a macrophage-mediated response to particulate debris of polyethylene, cement, or metal.[2] Osteolysis may occur in the presence of well-fixed or loose implants on either side of the joint.

Although there are no definitive, universal criteria for defining loose total hip implants, a change in implant position such as subsidence, the fracture of the cement mantle, or the fracture of the implant typically indicate that the component is loose. However, in some instances such as femoral impaction grafting for revision surgery, these criteria may not fully apply.

Gruen and colleagues identified four modes of mechanical failure of cemented femoral stems: pistoning, medial midstem pivot, calcar pivot, and cantilever bending.[3] They described seven zones around the femoral component that are to be assessed when classifying radiolucent lines or osteolysis (Diagram B). Radiolucency at the cement/bone interface occurs most commonly at the medial calcar (Zone 7), at the tip of the cement mantle (Zone 4), and along the proximal-lateral region (Zone 1). Radiolucencies on the initial postoperative film represent lack of penetration of the cement into the surrounding cancellous bone.

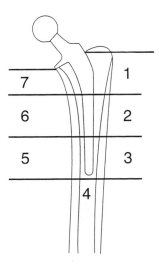

DIAGRAM B

Loosening of the cemented femoral component is defined as definite (migration of the component or cement), probable (a continuous radiolucent line around the entire cement mantle), or possible (a radiolucent line along more than 50% of the cement/bone interface.[4] Although a radiolucent line of more than 2 mm is suggestive of loosening, progression of the radiolucent line is more important. An intramedullary weightbearing pedestal sometimes forms adjacent to the tip of an uncemented femoral stem as a reaction to micromotion of the implant.

This finding suggests loosening but is not necessarily indicative of it. Stress shielding in the calcar suggests solid osteointegration of an uncemented femoral component.

We evaluate acetabular implants in several standard ways. The angles of the implant abduction and anteversion are measured and gaps at the implant/bone interface are documented. The ideal angle for abduction is 40 to 45 degrees as measured from a horizontal line drawn along the interischial line on the AP radiograph. The ideal angle for anteversion is usually 20 degrees. This is best assessed on a shoot-through lateral of the pelvis. The angles of abduction and anteversion may be purposefully varied within a fairly wide range, depending on anatomic or biomechanical factors assessed by the surgeon.

When the acetabular interface is evaluated, we usually report and quantify any gaps in contact along the periphery. Sometimes these gaps are true and sometimes they are only apparent. Gaps and focal osteolysis at the acetabular interface are classified according to the zones described by DeLee and Charnley.[5] Zone 1 is the lateral third, Zone 2 is the central third, and Zone 3 is the medial third (Diagram C). When lucency is present only in Zone 1, there is a 7% chance the implant will be loose at revision surgery. This figure increases to 71% when two zones show lucency. If there is a continuous radiolucent line around an acetabular implant, there is a 94% chance the implant is loose.[6]

Text continued on page 129

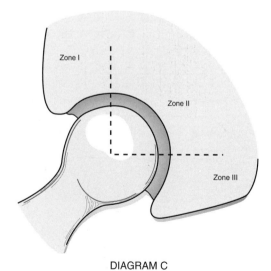

DIAGRAM C

FIGURE 6–1 In this bilateral hybrid total hip replacement, the acetabular component is cementless and there is an acetabular screw. The acetabular component on the right side is in 45 degrees of abduction. The acetabular component on the left side is in 60 degrees of abduction. Both femoral components are well cemented and are without any radiographic evidence of debonding. The collar-calcar contact is excellent. The acetabular interfaces are excellent and do not demonstrate any gaps. There is Grade 1 heterotopic ossification in the region of the iliopsoas tendon.[7]

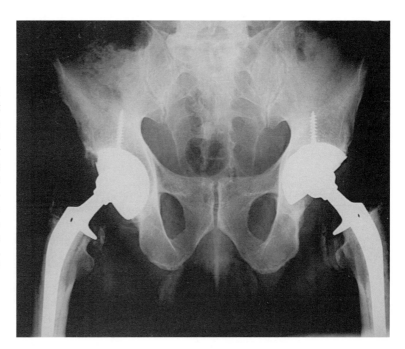

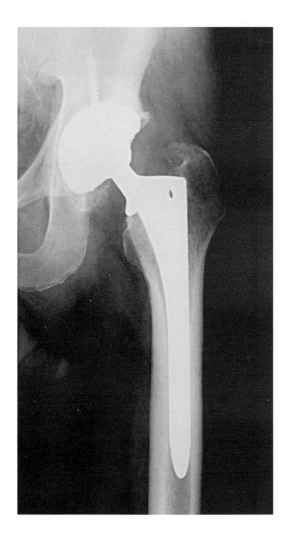

FIGURE 6–2 In this cementless total hip replacement, the acetabular component is in approximately 50 degrees of abduction and there is an acetabular screw that provides supplemental fixation. No acetabular gaps are seen and the interfaces between the implant and the bone are excellent. The femoral component is in neutral position (not in varus or valgus position), and there is excellent contact between the implant and the cortical bone of the femoral diaphysis. No osteolysis is present.

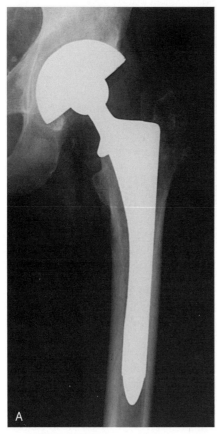

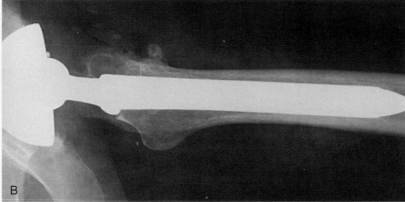

FIGURE 6–3   A: This is a 3-month postoperative AP radiograph of a ce-mentless total hip arthroplasty. The acetabular component is in 40 degrees of abduction, and the acetabular interfaces appear to be excellent. There is an apparent gap in Zone 2, but closer inspection reveals that there is trabecular bone right up to the implant. The acetabular component is minimally uncovered by host bone laterally. The femoral component is in neutral position and has excellent cortical contact within the femoral diaphysis. The collar-calcar contact is also good. There is no dislocation or fracture. **B:** This radiograph is a shoot-through lateral, the only radiograph by which acetabular component anteversion can be accurately measured. The acetabular implant is 10 degrees anteverted. On the femoral side, there is intimate bony apposition with the implant.

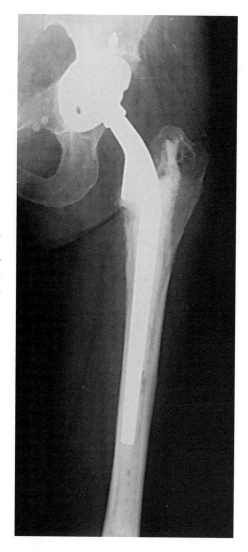

FIGURE 6–4 This hybrid revision has a femoral component that is a calcar replacement stem designed to replace proximal bone loss in the femur. Here it is used as a cemented implant in an elderly patient as treatment for a failed femoral component. The component is in slight valgus position and there is a cement void in Zone 3. The cementless acetabular component is in 50 degrees of abduction and is supplementally fixed with a single screw. The medial wall of the acetabulum is quite thin.

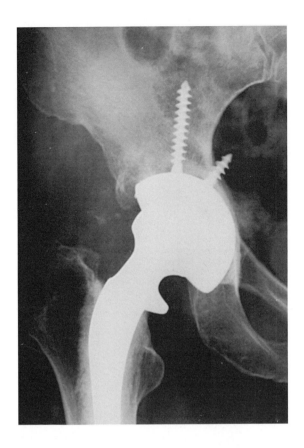

FIGURE 6–5 The patient in this figure has a cementless acetabular component and a cemented monoblock femoral component. The acetabular component is abducted 55 degrees (more vertical than is desirable), and there are acetabular screws. The most medial acetabular screw goes through the medial wall of the pelvis and into the sciatic notch. This position could cause sciatic nerve palsy, particularly if the screw were longer. The lucencies adjacent to the superior screw probably represent overlying bowel gas.

FIGURE 6–6 A and **B:** This patient sustained a displaced femoral neck fracture that was treated with a cemented hemiarthroplasty utilizing an anterolateral approach to the hip. Both views demonstrate that the endoprosthesis is located in the acetabulum. The cement technique is very good (Grade B), and there is good collar-calcar contact. There is Grade 1 heterotopic ossification superior and anterior to the greater trochanter, a typical finding when an anterolateral approach is used.

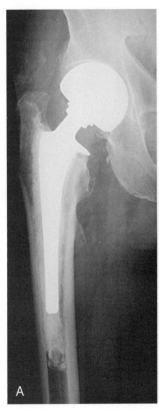

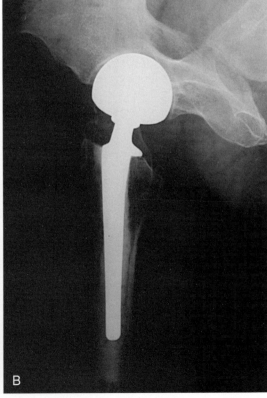

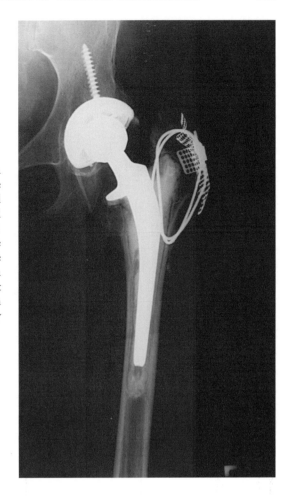

FIGURE 6–7 This is a hybrid revision total hip replacement. On the acetabular side, a titanium cementless cup is placed and a single screw is used for supplemental fixation. The cup is slightly uncovered laterally. The acetabular interfaces look excellent. On the femoral side, there is a cemented stem. The cement technique is a Grade C2 with a cement void seen medially. The radiolucent line around the cement mantle is evidence not of loosening but rather of incomplete cement penetration at the time of revision. The radiolucency seen at the tip of the femoral component is a distal centralizer made out of methyl methacrylate cement without barium. This lack of barium makes it appear radiolucent. The greater trochanter was extremely osteopenic and was fixed using two cables and Vitallium mesh.

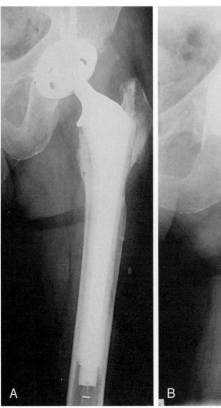
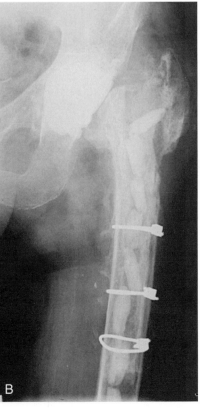

FIGURE 6–8 The treatment of an infected total hip replacement by implant removal utilizing an extended greater trochanteric osteotomy is demonstrated. **A:** In this hybrid total hip replacement, on the femoral side, there is bone loss beneath the greater trochanter where the patient had previous debridement. He had persistent infection that was treated by removing the implant and cement. Because of the extensive and high-quality cementing, an extended osteotomy was necessary to remove all of the cement. There is a slight radiolucent line around the cement column next to the cortical bone, but this is not evidence of loosening. This implant is well fixed. **B:** A healed extended greater trochanteric osteotomy is shown. There is a large piece of antibiotic-impregnated bone cement in the acetabulum and there are antibiotic beads in the femur. Three cables are visible; they were used to fix the osteotomy. Essentially, the lateral third of the femur was removed from the rest of the bone to create a large window that would facilitate the removal of the implant and cement. There are some small areas of heterotopic bone formation along the medial aspect of the femur that are typical of postoperative change.

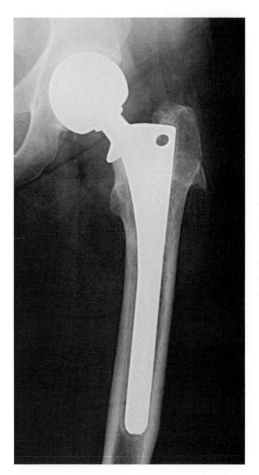

FIGURE 6–9   This loose, cementless unipolar hemiarthroplasty was performed for a displaced femoral neck fracture. The patient now presents with thigh pain. The femoral component shows several signs that indicate the presence of a loose implant, including a radiolucent line in Zones 1 and 4. The tip of the implant is up against the cortical bone laterally, and there is cortical hypertrophy at the tip. This is an example, in an older patient, of a press-fit implant that has settled into a slight varus position and has a very high likelihood of being loose. There are no definitive signs of loosening but several subtle signs that indicate that this is the likely cause of the patient's thigh pain.

FIGURE 6–10   This is a radiograph of a cemented total hip replacement utilizing an all-polyethylene acetabular component and a stainless steel, cemented monoblock femoral component. The femoral component has debonded and subsided, and is in valgus position. There is a large radiolucent space lateral to the proximal portion of the implant where it has debonded from the cement in Zone 1, and it has also debonded in Zone 4. A cement fracture is marked with an arrow. This femoral component is definitely loose, based on this radiographic appearance. The acetabular component demonstrates evidence of polyethylene wear, and there is a radiolucent line in Zones 2 and 3.

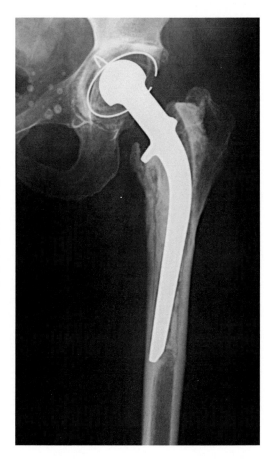

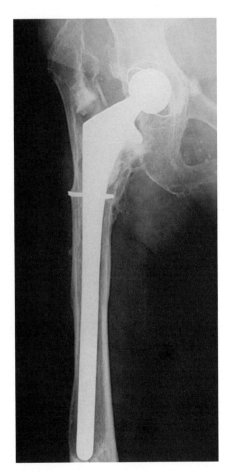

FIGURE 6–11   This is another example of a loose femoral component. At the time of revision it was found to have been cemented proximally and press-fit distally. A cerclage wire was used to fix a cortical strut allograft that had become incorporated. There is massive debonding proximally, and the stem has subsided from the location revealed in previous films. Distally, there is a substantial osteolytic lesion around the tip of the implant and thinning of the lateral cortical bone. This patient is at risk for pathologic femur fracture. The acetabular component is a cemented all-polyethylene cup that demonstrates eccentric wear.

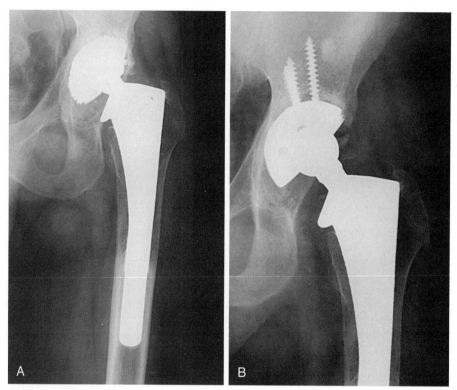

FIGURE 6–12   A: A loose acetabular component is visible on this radiograph of a long-term follow-up. The implant was tightly fitted into the pelvis, and screws were used to fix the modular polyethylene to the metal shell. There is a radiolucent line around the entire cup, and the patient had groin pain. On the femoral side, there is extensive bony ingrowth into the distal aspect of the porous coating, densification distally, and stress shielding proximally. The fact that the collar of the implant does not have contact with the femur is inconsequential in this radiograph, as the prosthesis was inserted to that depth intentionally. Further insertion of the implant at the time of surgery might have caused a fracture. Cementless femoral implants often cannot be inserted until there is collar-calcar contact. **B:** The acetabular implant has been revised; it is now a cementless component using acetabular screw fixation. The three screws are in the ilium. The femoral stem was well fixed and not revised, but the femoral head was exchanged to facilitate acetabular exposure.

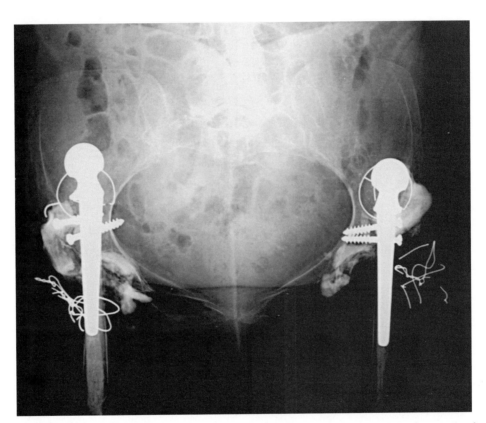

FIGURE 6–13 This radiograph demonstrates complete bilateral dislocation of a cemented total hip replacement. Both trochanters had been fixed using wire that has since fragmented. Both acetabular components have come completely loose and have migrated. The screws were used to fix an allograft femoral head to the ilium to supplement the acetabular bone stock. The metal rings near the femoral heads are marker rings in the polyethylene liner of the acetabular component.

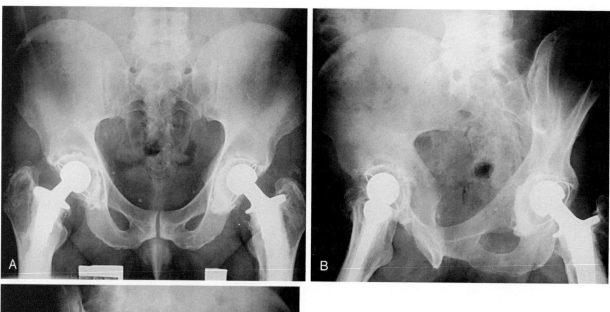

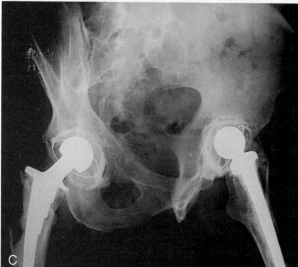

FIGURE 6–14 This series of radiographs demonstrates loosening of bilateral cemented acetabular implants. **A:** In the AP view of the pelvis, a large radiolucent line around both acetabular components is seen. There is eccentric polyethylene wear that is more pronounced on the right. **B** and **C:** There is a complete radiolucent line in both Judet views. With a complete radiolucent demarcation of the socket, there is a 94% chance of finding the implant loose at reoperation. Osteolysis is evident in both greater trochanters.

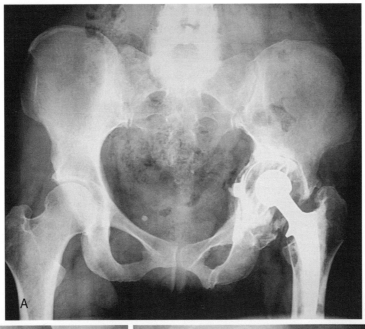

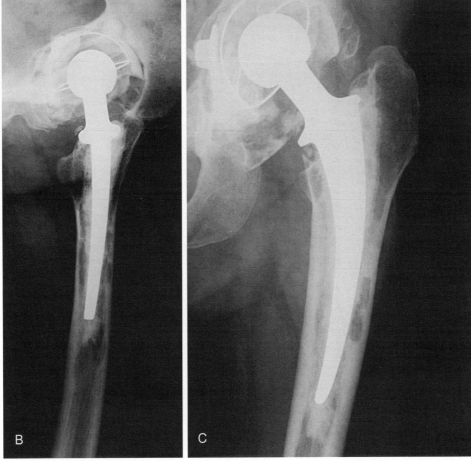

FIGURE 6–15   A, B, and **C:** This is an 18-year-old cemented total hip replacement that demonstrates a complete radiolucent line around the acetabular implant and osteolysis in all three acetabular zones. It appears that the acetabular implant has migrated superiorly and medially approximately 1.5 cm from the original postoperative position, and protrusio is now evident. The femoral implant is a monoblock type (the femoral head is not modular). The AP and lateral views of the proximal femur demonstrate that the femoral implant has debonded. There is substantial intracortical osteolysis visible in both views, and there is an osteolytic lesion 1 cm distal to the tip of the femoral implant that is best seen on the lateral view. The cortical osteolysis is pronounced near regions of C2 defects in the bone cement. This debonding is radiographic evidence of a loose stem.

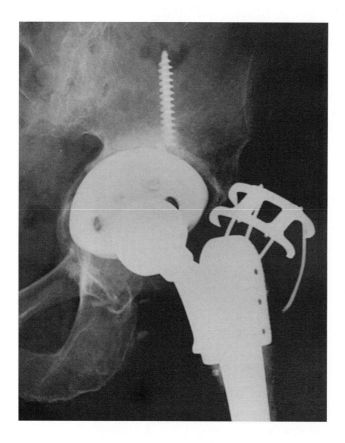

FIGURE 6–16 This radiograph demonstrates a cementless titanium acetabular component that was fixed by press-fitting and supplemental screws. There is a complete radiolucent line around the implant and an acetabular screw has broken, so the component should be considered loose. The greater trochanter fixation has also failed, as there is a broken cable and migration of the grip device. The femoral implant is a calcar replacement stem.

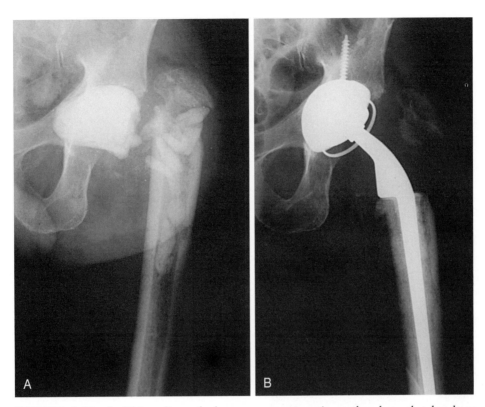

FIGURE 6–17 A: This radiograph demonstrates a resection arthroplasty that has been used to treat a chronically infected total hip replacement. There is a large antibiotic-impregnated cement spacer in the acetabulum, and there are cement beads in the proximal femur. The greater trochanter has been fractured and is completely separate from the proximal femur. **B:** Because of the extensive muscle loss around the hip and the trochanter fracture, a hybrid total hip replacement with a constrained acetabular liner was chosen for stability. This constrained liner locks the femoral head into the acetabulum and is very effective in preventing dislocation. Although short-term results are good, the theoretical disadvantages of constrained liners are an increased rate of wear due to thinner polyethylene and the fact that dislocation may still occur as a result of impingement. The radiograph shows a cementless acetabular implant, and the locking ring can be seen capturing the femoral head. The femoral component is a cemented calcar replacement stem that was necessary in order to gain the necessary length and offset for stability.

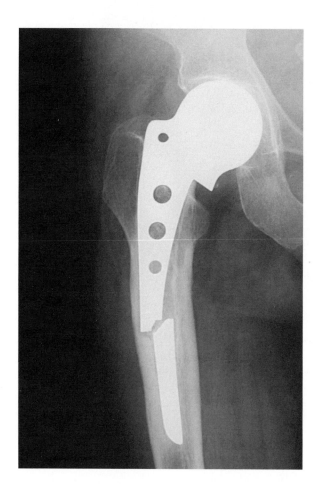

FIGURE 6–18 This is a cementless, unipolar, stainless steel femoral component. Fatigue fracture of the stem has occurred secondary to cantilever bending in the presence of poor proximal and good distal fixation.

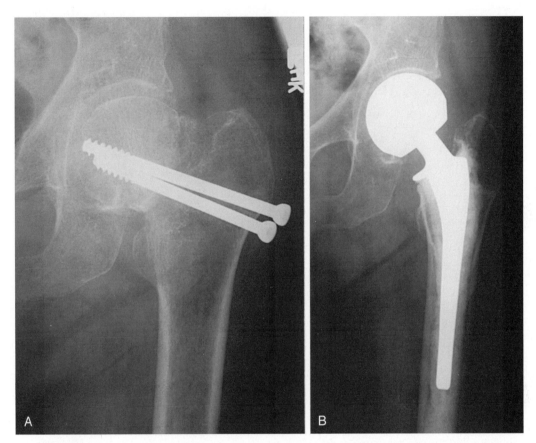

FIGURE 6–19   A: This radiograph shows two 6.5-mm cannulated screws that were used to fix a displaced femoral neck fracture. The fracture has collapsed into varus malalignment, and the screws have backed out as the fracture has collapsed. The patient had pain with ambulation, and persistent lucency at the fracture site suggests that a nonunion is present. **B:** This radiograph demonstrates a cemented unipolar hemiarthroplasty. The acetabular implant is located and sized appropriately. The stem is centralized both proximally and distally. The radiolucency between the cement and the bone represents incomplete penetration of the cancellous bone by the cement at the time of implantation but is not evidence of loosening.

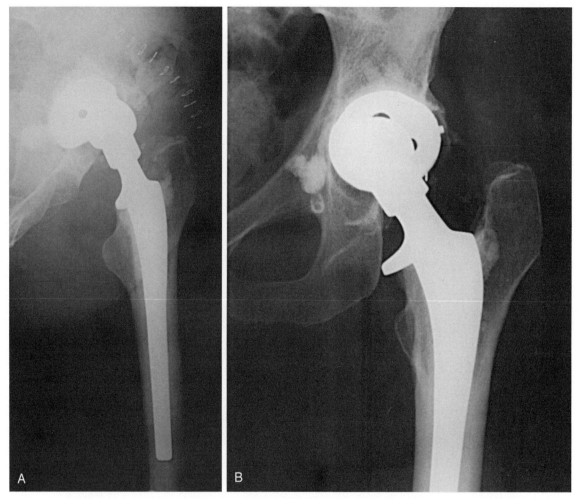

FIGURE 6–20 A: This AP radiograph, taken immediately after surgery, demonstrates subluxation of the femoral head in a cemented total hip arthroplasty. The femoral head is not located within the acetabular implant, but it is difficult to tell if this is a true dislocation or a subluxation. **B:** This AP radiograph, in which the patient is in a hip abduction orthosis, demonstrates the absence of concentric alignment of the femoral head in the acetabular implant. Anteversion of the acetabular implant is difficult to assess on an AP radiograph, but the fact that one can see right through the screw holes suggests that the cup is excessively anteverted.

FIGURE 6–20 *Continued.* **C:** This is a true shoot-through lateral taken when the patient was in a brace. The acetabular implant is anteverted approximately 70 degrees. Malposition of the acetabular implant leaves the femoral head uncovered anteriorly, which accounts for the instability. This patient required acetabular revision with less anteversion of the component to provide stability.

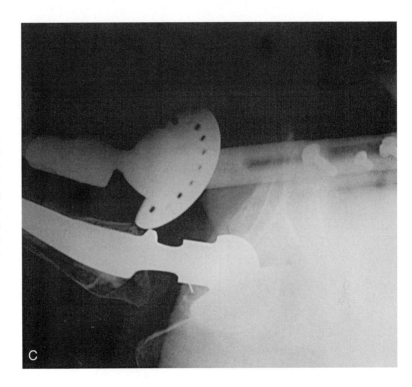

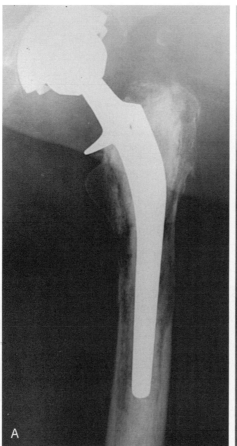
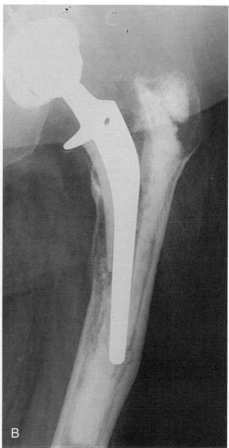
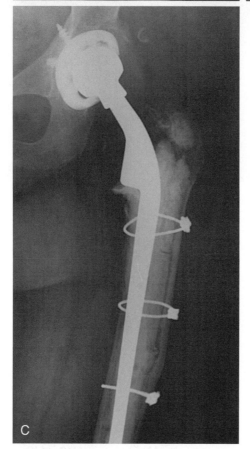

FIGURE 6–21 A: This is an early post-operative radiograph of a hybrid total hip replacement. Poor cement technique has left voids in Zones 2 and 4 (Grade C2). There also appears to be an osteolytic lesion in Zone 2. Around the proximal lateral aspect of the femoral implant (Zone 1), there appears to be debonding of the cement from the implant. **B:** This radiograph taken after 1 year demonstrates massive debonding of the implant and multiple cement fractures. There may be a pathologic fracture in Zone 5 of the femur in the area of osteolysis below the lesser trochanter. **C:** Because this patient was older and had low activity demands, she underwent revision to a cemented stem. An extended trochanteric osteotomy was performed to fully expose the proximal femur, and a calcar replacement long stem was cemented. Cables were used to secure the osteotomy, which appears healed. Some areas of cement, such as that seen in the greater trochanter, could be left behind because there was no evidence of infection.

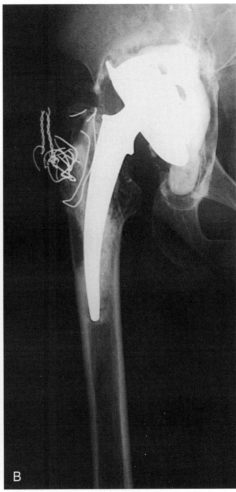

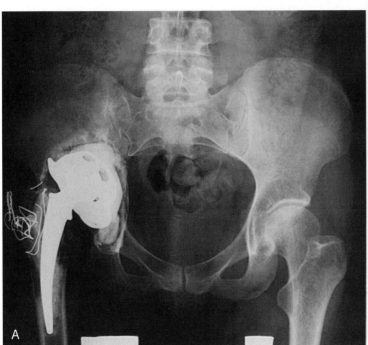

FIGURE 6–22 A and **B:** These radiographs demonstrate the long-term sequelae of a cemented total hip replacement in a patient with severe acetabular dysplasia. The acetabular implant is a cemented antiprotrusio shell with a cemented, all-polyethylene liner, one of the first metal shells designed for severe protrusio. There is a complete radiolucent line around the acetabular implant on the AP pelvis (A) and Judet (B) views. This implant is loose. On the femoral side there are broken wires left from the reattachment of the greater trochanter. However, the greater trochanter osteotomy has healed. There is osteolysis around the femoral implant in Zones 1 and 2. There is also osteolysis in the lesser trochanter. The femoral implant has debonded in Zones 1 and 4 and is loose, based on radiographic appearance.

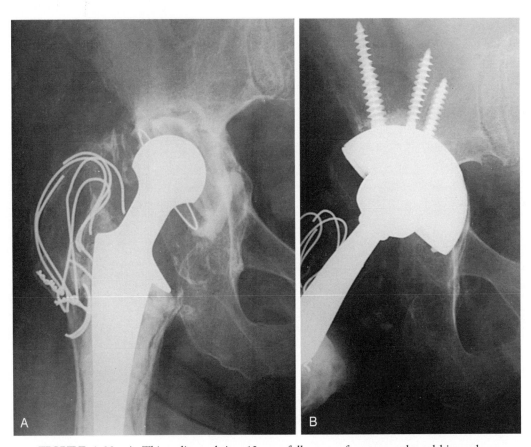

FIGURE 6–23   A: This radiograph is a 12-year follow-up of a cemented total hip replacement that used a greater trochanter osteotomy for exposure. The acetabular implant has a
large radiolucent line in this view and in the two oblique views of the pelvis (not shown). It
has changed position, which is definitive evidence of a loose implant. There is eccentric wear,
with the head resting superiorly in the polyethylene liner. The greater trochanter osteotomy
has united, although the wires are broken. This is a common finding. Although there is a
discontinuous radiolucent line in Zones 1 and 7, the femoral implant is not loose. Grade 1
heterotopic ossification is present. **B:** This figure demonstrates a revision to hybrid total hip
replacement. The acetabular implant is in 40 degrees of abduction. Four screws were used in
the ilium to supplement fixation. A defect in the medial wall may be present but is difficult
to assess on this view. The femoral implant has been revised to a cemented calcar replacement stem.

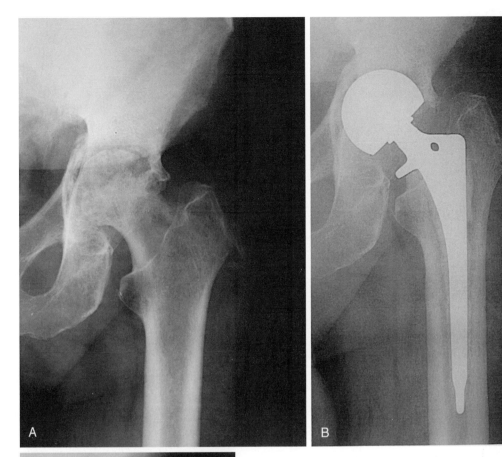

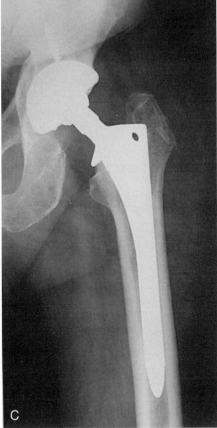

FIGURE 6–24   **A:** This radiograph shows the hip joint of a patient who has had chronic osteomyelitis of the femoral head and acetabulum. The patient presented with an infected hip joint and was treated by arthrotomy and debridement. However, he developed chronic osteomyelitis, which was managed in two stages. **B:** A unipolar PROSTALAC was placed after excision of the femoral head and debridement of the acetabulum and pelvis. This implant is coated with cement that contains antibiotics, a technique that produces high local antibiotic concentration without causing systemic side effects. The prosthesis is implanted loosely, as a temporary spacer. Weightbearing is allowed. **C:** During the second stage of the procedure, the PROSTALAC is removed and a new implant is placed. In this radiograph, a cementless total hip replacement is seen. The acetabular implant is in 40 degrees of abduction, and a single acetabular screw is used for supplemental fixation. The cup may not be contacting the medial wall, but because of medial deficiency, the implant was press-fitted between the anterior and posterior columns of the pelvis. The femoral implant is a cementless femoral stem. There is excellent cortical contact distally and excellent collar-calcar contact proximally.

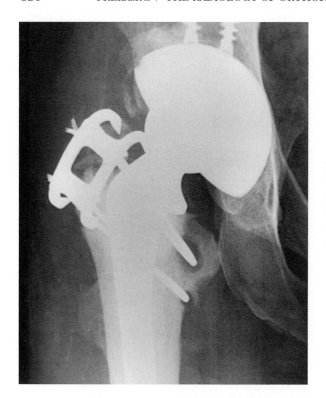

FIGURE 6–25 One of the possible long-term changes around a loose cable is shown in this radiograph. Osteolysis in the lesser trochanter and in the subtrochanteric region has resulted from motion of the fixation device. The cables show fretting, which can contribute to third-body wear of the polyethylene liner.

FIGURE 6–26 This is a cementless total hip replacement with modular femoral and acetabular components. **A:** The femoral component is well fixed, and excellent proximal bony ingrowth has occurred around the porous pads. **B:** The acetabular implant shows a locking screw that has backed out, and the polyethylene was found to be loose at revision surgery.

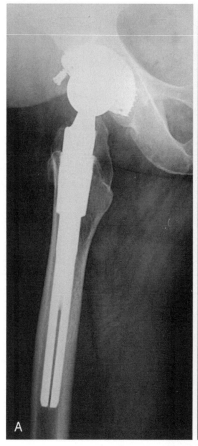

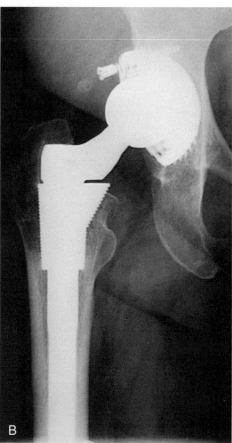

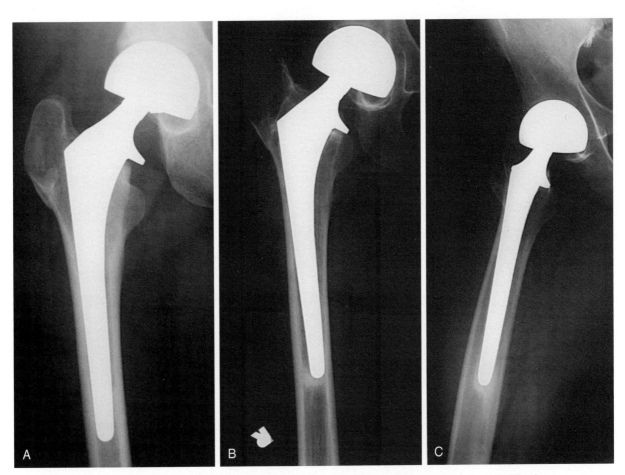

FIGURE 6–27 A: This radiograph demonstrates the excellent proximal fit and fill of a cementless bipolar hemiarthroplasty, but there is no porous ingrowth surface. **B:** At 5 years, the femoral component has subsided, with resorption of the calcar region. It has moved into varus alignment, and there is a radiodense pedestal around the tip of the implant, which is consistent with a loose femoral component. **C:** This lateral radiograph shows the pedestal, which is a reaction to micromotion at the tip of the stem. Pedestal formation is suggestive of a loose implant but is not pathognomonic for loosening.

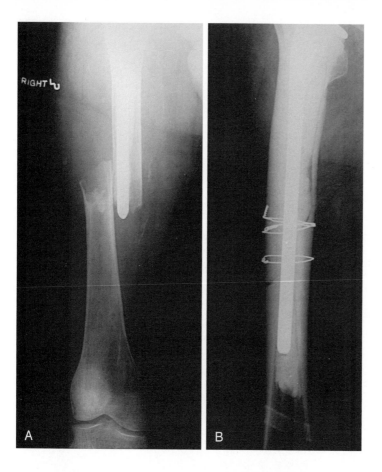

FIGURE 6–28   A: This radiograph shows a cemented femoral implant with a periprosthetic femur fracture. There is rarefaction around the tip of the stem that is consistent with a previously diagnosed osteolytic lesion. The femoral implant was loose on other views and at the time of revision surgery. B: A femoral cortical window was made for removal of the cement, and the implant was tapped out from below. This radiograph shows the cemented revision. Several 18-gauge stainless steel wires were used to hold the cortical window in place. There is incomplete cement filling medially, but the cement technique is otherwise excellent. For periprosthetic fractures, the tip of the revision stem should usually bypass the fracture by at least two cortical diameters.

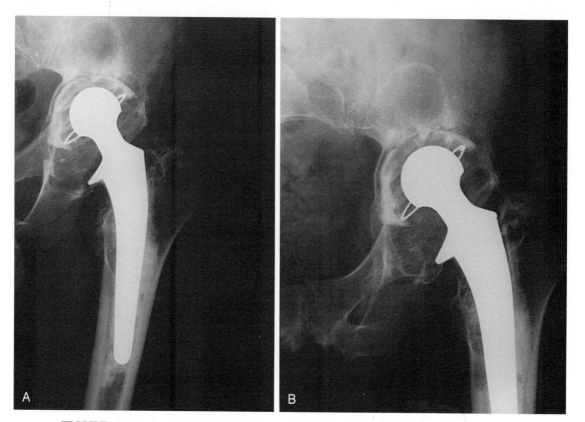

FIGURE 6–29   A and B: This is an 8-year follow-up radiograph of a cemented total hip replacement that demonstrates proximal femoral osteolysis caused by debris resulting from polyethylene wear. There is also a 3-cm cyst in the ilium that was found to contain polyethylene debris at revision surgery.

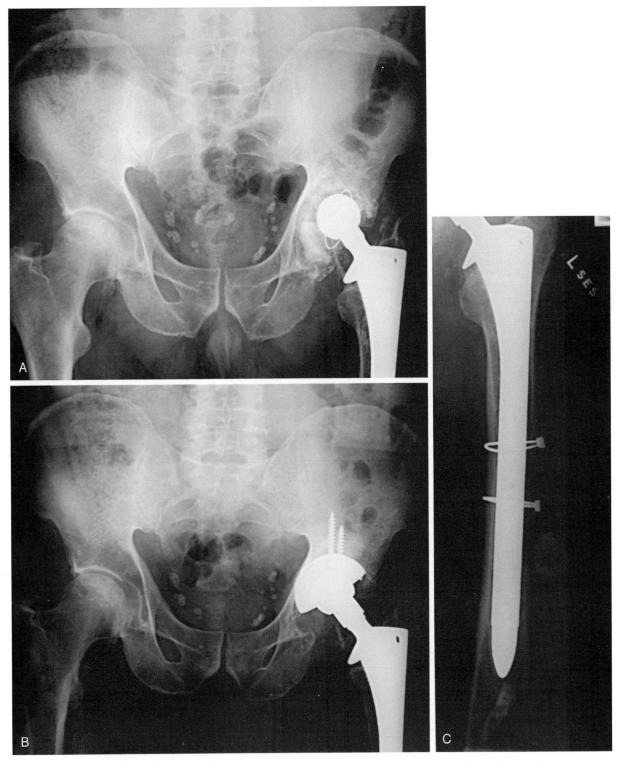

FIGURE 6–30 A: This acetabular component has changed position, and osteolysis and cement fracture are present. There is also radiographic evidence of eccentric polyethylene wear. At the time of revision surgery both implants were found to be loose and both were revised. **B:** The acetabulum was revised to a cementless acetabular component, and the femoral component was revised to a cementless long stem. **C:** The cables on the femur were used to close a femoral cortical window that facilitated cement removal.

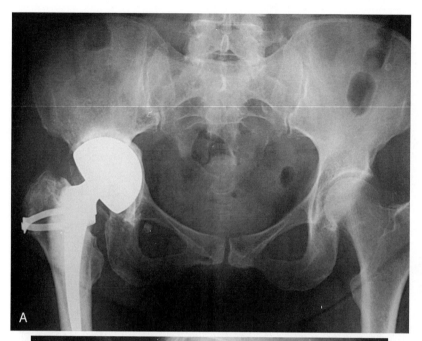

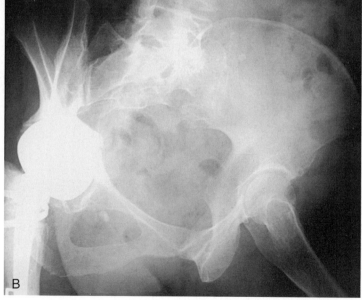

FIGURE 6–31 A: This AP radiograph shows a revision hip replacement with a cemented femoral component and a large bipolar acetabular implant. The implant has migrated with time, as evidenced by acetabular protrusio. The patient had debilitating groin pain caused by acetabular cartilage wear. **B:** The medial wall is intact but thin.

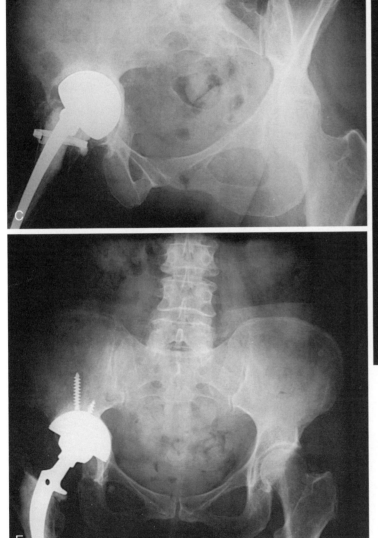

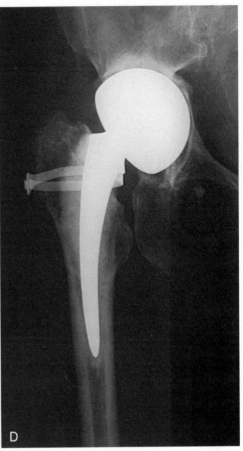

FIGURE 6–31 *Continued.* **C:** As in **B,** the medial wall is intact but thin. **D:** The femoral component was debonded and loose. **E:** The implants were revised. At revision, the acetabulum was converted to a cementless acetabular component with supplemental screws and medial bone graft.

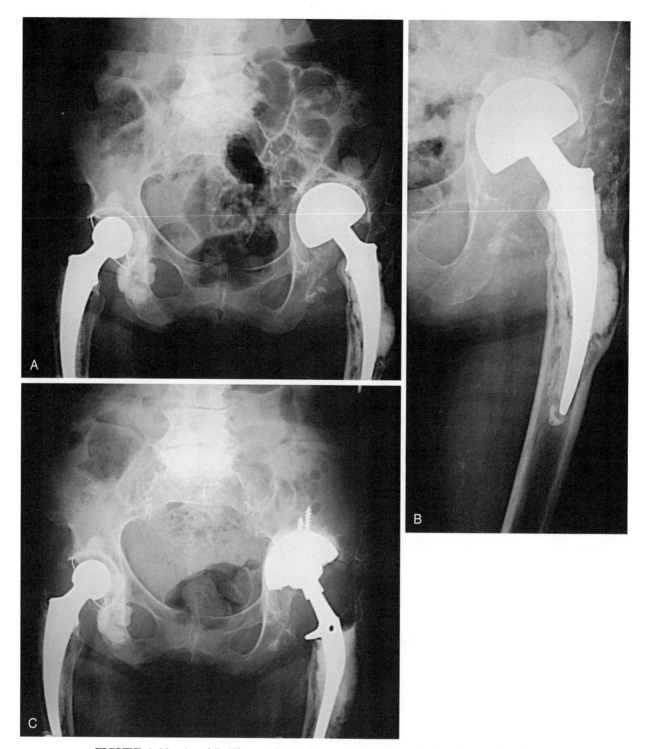

FIGURE 6–32 A and **B**: These radiographs reveal massive osteolysis in the proximal femur around a cemented implant. The bipolar implant is loose in the acetabulum, and this appearance could be consistent with either septic or aseptic loosening. **C:** The implant was revised to a cementless acetabular component with bone graft and a long cemented femoral component. A high hip center was used for acetabular reconstruction. (To create a high hip center, the center of the hip's rotation is placed more than 3 cm above a line drawn between the obturator foramina.)

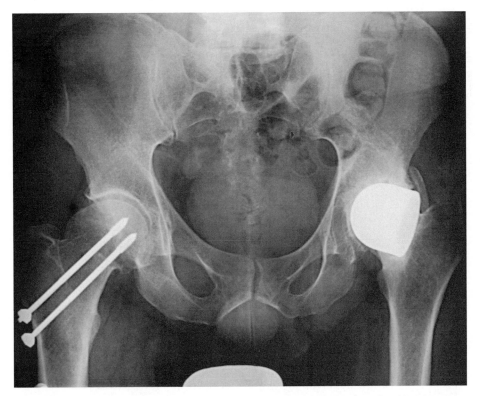

FIGURE 6–33   This radiograph shows a loose cup arthroplasty. In the other hip, the patient has two Knowles pins that were used to treat slipped capital femoral epiphysis in childhood.

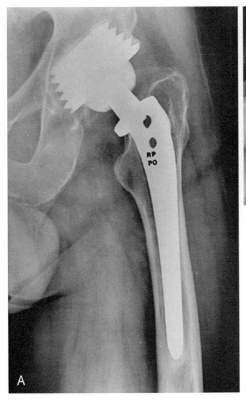

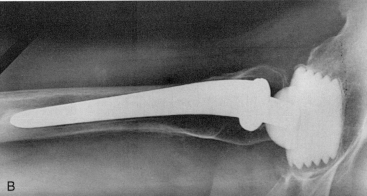

FIGURE 6–34   A and **B:** An AP and a lateral view show the long-term follow-up of a Mittelmier ceramic-on-ceramic total hip replacement. There are subtle radiolucencies around the acetabular and femoral components, but the reconstruction is not painful and the patient has good function. (Courtesy of Dr. Thomas P. Schmalzried, Los Angeles, CA)

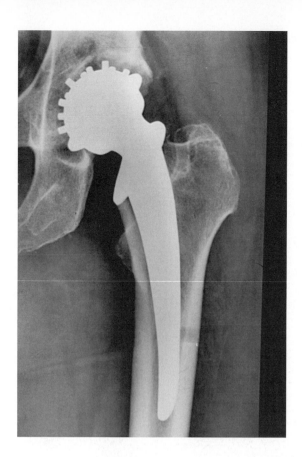

FIGURE 6–35 This radiograph is a long-term follow-up of a McKee-Farrar metal-on-metal prosthesis. The femoral and acetabular components are cementless, and there is no polyethylene in the articulation. The entire hip replacement is made of cobalt-chrome. (Courtesy of Dr. Thomas P. Schmalzried, Los Angeles, CA)

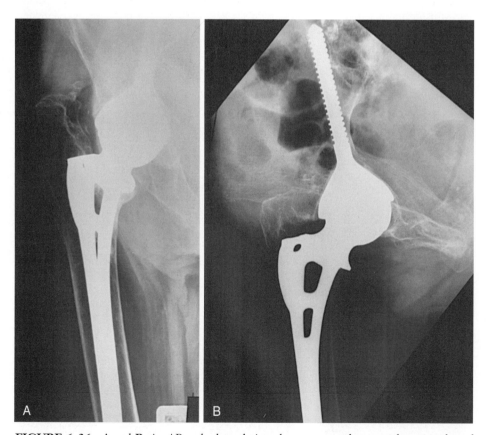

FIGURE 6–36 A and B: An AP and a lateral view show a cementless, metal-on-metal total hip replacement that uses a large acetabular screw to effect acetabular fixation. The fenestrated areas in the femoral component allow bone ingrowth around the implant, fixing it to the proximal femur. (Courtesy of Dr. Thomas P. Schmalzried, Los Angeles, CA)

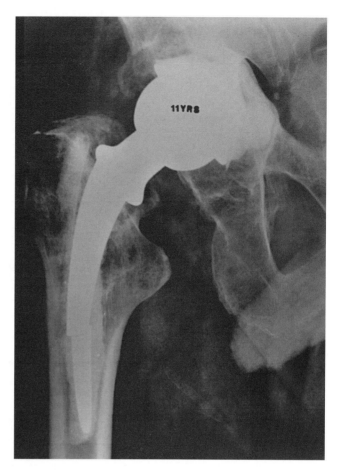

FIGURE 6–37 This radiograph is an example of a failed metal-on-metal Mueller prosthesis. Both implants are cemented implants. There is acetabular and femoral osteolysis and the femoral component is loose and fractured. The acetabular component has a complete radiolucent line around it and has moved from the position shown on previous radiographs; thus, it is loose. (Courtesy of Dr. Thomas P. Schmalzried, Los Angeles, CA.)

REFERENCES

1. Barrack RL, Mulroy RD, Harris WH. Improved cementing techniques and femoral component loosening in young patients with hip arthroplasty: a 12-year radiographic review. J Bone Joint Surg 1992;74B:385–389.
2. Jasty MJ, Floyd WE, Schiller AL, et al. Localized osteolysis in stable, nonseptic total hip replacement. J Bone Joint Surg 1986;68A:912–919.
3. Gruen TA, McNeice GM, Amstutz HC. "Modes of failure" of cemented stem-type femoral components: a radiographic analysis of loosening. Clin Orthop 1979;141:16–27.
4. Harris WH, McCarthy JC, O'Neill DA. Femoral component loosening using contemporary techniques of femoral cement fixation. J Bone Joint Surg 1982;64A:1063–1067.
5. DeLee JG, Charnley J. Radiological demarcation of cemented sockets in total hip replacement. Clin Orthop 1976;121:20–32.
6. Hodgkinson JP, Shelley P, Wroblewski BM. The correlation between the roentgenographic appearance and operative findings at the bone-cement junction of the socket in Charnley low-friction arthroplasties. Clin Orthop 1988;228:105–109.
7. Brooker AF, Bowerman JW, Robinson RA, et al. Ectopic ossification following total hip replacement: incidence and a method of classification. J Bone Joint Surg 1973;55A:1629–1632.
8. Goetz DD, Capello WN, Callaghan JJ, et al. Salvage of total hip instability with a constrained acetabular component. Clin Orthop 1998;355:171–181.
9. Duncan CP, Beauchamp C. A temporary antibiotic-loaded joint replacement system for management of complex infections involving the hip. Orthop Clin North Am 1993;24:751–759.

7

—

Impaction Allografting with Cement for Femoral Component Revision

SETH S. LEOPOLD

AARON G. ROSENBERG

The views expressed in this chapter are those of the authors and do not reflect the official policy of the Department of Defense of the United States Government.

Revision hip arthroplasty in the setting of severe femoral bone-stock deficiency is one of the most challenging and controversial problems in hip arthroplasty. Proximal femoral replacement arthroplasty has been advocated as one possible solution, but high rates of dislocation and infection have been seen with endoprostheses of this type. Allograft-prosthetic composite reconstructions using massive proximal femoral bulk grafts have been used in an attempt to reconstitute missing bone stock, but issues of nonunion, graft resorption, and infection have resulted in limited enthusiasm for this technique.

Extensively porous-coated, cementless femoral implants are now in common use, and excellent results have been reported with them at long-term follow-up. These implants typically bypass the deficient proximal femoral metaphysis to obtain stability with distal press-fit and eventual diaphyseal bone ingrowth; however, concerns remain about the fate of the relatively unloaded proximal femoral bone stock. Severe stress shielding and proximal bone atrophy have been observed with these implants (Fig. 7–1).

Impaction allografting with cement provides a potential alternative in these severely bone-deficient femurs. This technique seeks to provide a stable and durable femoral reconstruction while concurrently addressing the bone-stock deficiency.

The technique of femoral impaction allografting, as described by some workers, begins with removal of the loose stem and meticulous debridement of the remaining endosteum. Cortical defects must be contained with wire mesh or allograft struts. A distal canal restrictor is placed, and a neutrally aligned guide rod is threaded into it. The canal is packed tightly with fresh-frozen cancellous allograft, and increasingly larger cannulated tamps, shaped to resemble the femoral implant, are impacted into the allograft. Through repetitive packing of allograft and tamp impaction, a so-called neoendosteum is created; its walls consist of densely packed bone graft contained within the remaining cortical bone. Finally, the femoral prosthesis is cemented into the neoendosteum using contemporary cement techniques.

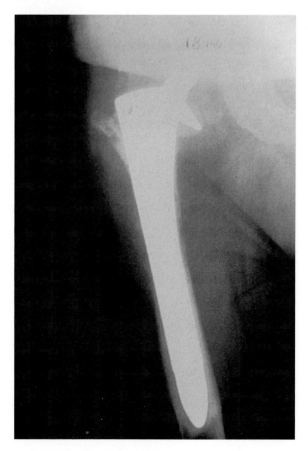

FIGURE 7–1 This extensively porous-coated revision femoral stem (Solution; Depuy, Warsaw, IN) depends upon diaphyseal press-fit for stability. Although it is easily ingrown and mechanically stable, fixation of this type often does not load the proximal femur. Severe stress shielding and proximal femoral bone loss can result, as seen in this patient 18 months postoperatively.

Impaction allografting can be time-consuming, technically demanding, and expensive; however, published radiographic and clinical success rates have ranged from 88 to 97% at short- to intermediate-term follow-up. Biopsy and retrieval studies have demonstrated that large areas of the graft indeed heal, and the technique can provide a stable reconstruction with an impressive amount of graft remodelling and even cortical reconstitution (Fig. 7–2). The long-term durability of femoral revisions performed with impaction allografting is not known.

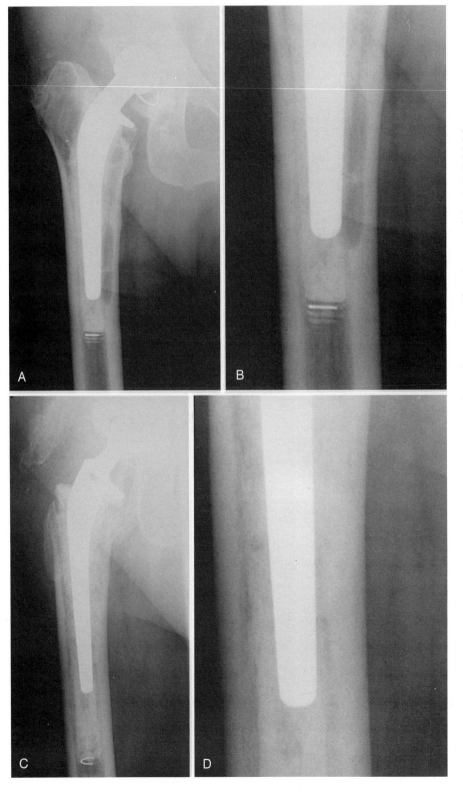

FIGURE 7–2 **A:** This antero-posterior (AP) hip radiograph in a 70-year-old man demonstrates an aseptically loose cemented femoral stem (6032 prosthesis; Zimmer, Warsaw, IN). This device includes a titanium-bearing surface and a 32-mm femoral head. Loosening of this implant is characteristically accompanied by cortical thinning and osteolysis, as is shown here. **B:** This detail from a preoperative radiograph demonstrates a large osteolytic lesion at the stem tip and thinning of the medial cortex. **C:** The hip was reconstructed using femoral impaction allografting with a precoated femoral stem (Harris Precoat; Zimmer). At 36 months postoperatively, the graft appears radiographically to be incorporated, and there is cortical healing of the osteolytic lesion. Migration of a greater trochanteric osteotomy is observed; this complication is present in up to 50% of patients undergoing impaction grafting when the transtrochanteric approach is used. **D:** A detail from the 36-month postoperative radiograph indicates that the osteolytic lesion seen on the preoperative radiograph appears to have healed, and the cortex has remodeled.

Complications of this technique include a rate of iatrogenic femoral fracture and perforation as high as 24% (Fig. 7–3), trochanteric nonunion in up to 50% of patients treated with the transtrochanteric approach, and stem subsidence in 8 to 44% of cases. The significance of stem subsidence is controversial and implant-dependent; some investigators have hypothesized that subsidence of a polished wedge-shaped stem will result in a beneficial compressive load on the bone graft, whereas others have associated subsidence with thigh pain, inequality of limb length, and prosthetic dislocation.

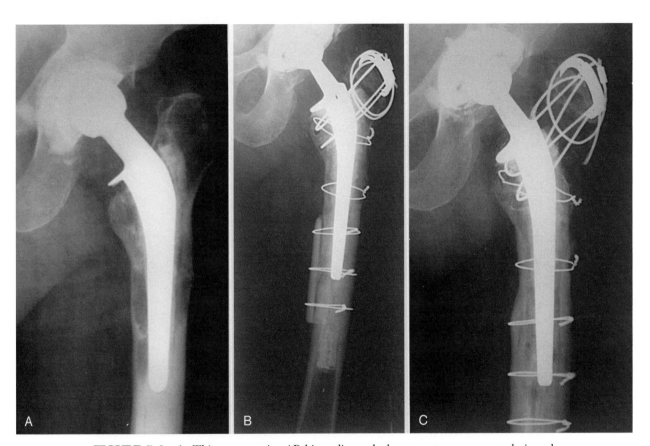

FIGURE 7–3   A: This preoperative AP hip radiograph demonstrates severe osteolysis and bone loss in the metaphyseal and diaphyseal regions around an aseptically loose cemented titanium femoral stem (6032 prosthesis; Zimmer). The preoperative Harris hip score was 51 out of 100 (poor). **B:** This radiograph, taken 6 weeks postoperatively, illustrates two common complications of impaction allografting: femoral perforation and migration of the greater trochanteric osteotomy. The perforation was noted intraoperatively and was treated with a medial cortical strut allograft and cerclage wires, and the greater trochanter was treated nonoperatively. **C:** At 71 months postoperatively, there is visible healing of the cortical strut allograft. The stem is stable and does not appear to have subsided. The greater trochanter migrated cephalad but stabilized over the first postoperative year at the location seen here. The patient has no pain or limitations referable to this reconstruction and had a Harris hip score of 81 (good).

Several femoral implant designs have been used for this procedure; the group that described the technique recommends a polished, double-tapered, wedge-shaped stem (Fig. 7–4). Stems with different geometries and surface finishes (Fig. 7–5) have been used, and the effect of stem design is just one of many known variables of this technique that still remain to be tested clinically.

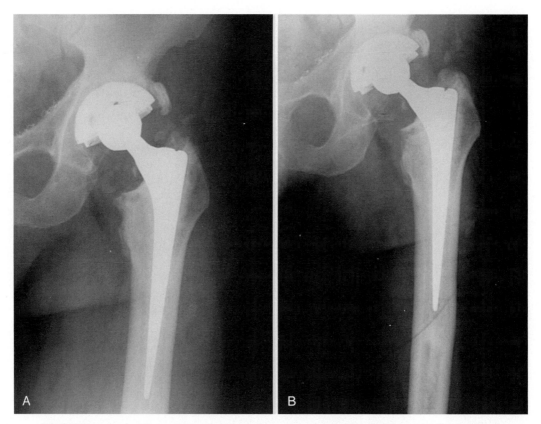

FIGURE 7–4   A: The technique of femoral impaction allografting, when initially described, used a highly polished, wedge-shaped implant with a biplanar taper, similar to the CPT stem (Collarless Polished Taper; Zimmer) shown here at 8 weeks postoperatively. This implant's design and surface finish may permit some stem subsidence without symptomatic loosening. Such subsidence may occur through cold flow of the cement mantle and may provide a beneficial compressive load on the cancellous graft. **B:** The femoral component has subsided about 2 mm (the radiolucency at the superolateral edge of the stem may be seen), but the Harris hip score is 90 (excellent) and the patient has no pain in that hip 50 months after revision. The appearance of the graft is characterized as stable (neither resorbed nor obviously incorporated).

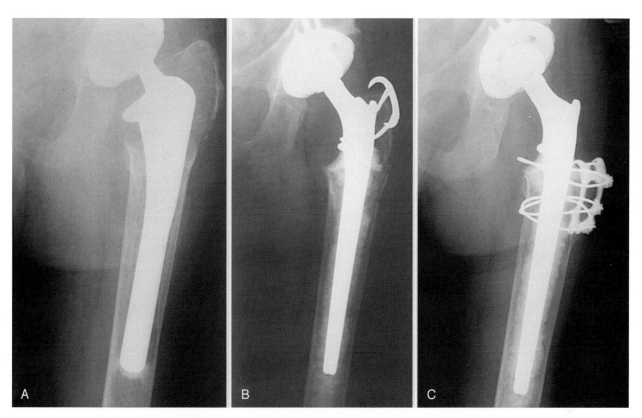

FIGURE 7–5   A: This preoperative radiograph demonstrates cortical thinning and significant widening of the intramedullary canal in a 53-year-old patient with ankylosing spondylitis. There is osteolysis at the tip of this first-generation cementless stem (Harris-Galante prosthesis; Zimmer), and the proximal bone-stock compromise has resulted in fracture of the greater trochanter. This case illustrates several of the important indications for impaction allografting: diaphyseal widening that would require a stem greater than 22 mm in diameter if cementless fixation were to be used, severe cortical thinning with osteolysis, and young age. The goals of the procedure include pain relief, durable fixation, and bone-stock reconstitution; the latter is particularly important for younger patients. **B:** Impaction allografting was performed using a cobalt-chrome stem that is tapered but is also roughened and normalized (6050 Calcar Replacement Stem; Osteonics, Allendale, NJ). Contrast this to the wedge-shaped, polished-taper stem shown in Figure 7–4. This AP hip radiograph, taken 6 weeks postoperatively, demonstrates a neutrally aligned stem and a cable-grip reattaching the greater trochanter to the shoulder of the implant and to the bone-deficient proximal femur. **C:** Severe proximal femoral bone deficiency resulted in a symptomatic greater trochanteric nonunion, which was treated with advancement and reattachment, shown here 29 months postoperatively. The endosteal graft appears to be stable, the stem has not subsided, and the greater trochanter has united in the more distal location. The patient's Harris hip score is 83 (good).

8

—

Measurement of Polyethylene Wear in Total Hip Joint Replacement

—

PETER A. DEVANE

J. GEOFFREY HORNE

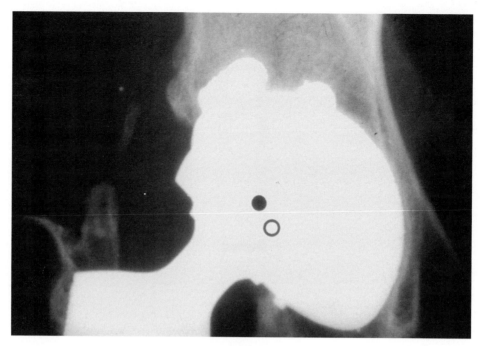

FIGURE 8–1

Central to this chapter is the inadequacy of many of the techniques available for the measurement of polyethylene wear in the acetabular components of total hip joint replacement (THJR). As a result of beam scatter caused by implanted metal, sophisticated imaging modalities such as computerized tomography and magnetic resonance imaging cannot be used. Thus, investigators are dependent on plane radiographs for the measurement of polyethylene wear (Fig. 8–1).

Uniradiographic and Duoradiographic Techniques

Uniradiographic and *duoradiographic* are the terms used by Clarke and colleagues to describe techniques first developed by Charnley to determine the rate of polyethylene wear in THJR.[1] Although several reports on the effect of femoral head size[2] and polyethylene wear debris[3] had appeared in the late 1960s, the first method of measuring wear based on plane radiographs was developed by Charnley and Cupic in 1973 (Fig. 8–2).[4] The uniradiographic technique used only the most recent anteroposterior (AP) radiograph to measure polyethylene thickness, but with criticism, the methodology was modified to incorporate the thickness of the plastic in the postoperative film at the same point. This was later termed the duoradiographic technique.[5] All measurements were scaled for the known size of the femoral head. Accuracy was reported as plus or minus 0.5 mm. Measurement of 69 hips, with an average 9-year follow-up, provided a mean linear wear rate of 0.15 mm per year. Based on an assessment of the reproducibility of the duoradiographic technique, Clarke and colleagues found that resulting errors were of the same order as the wear magnitudes being measured and concluded that wear measurements could not be made on the basis of clinical radiographs.[6]

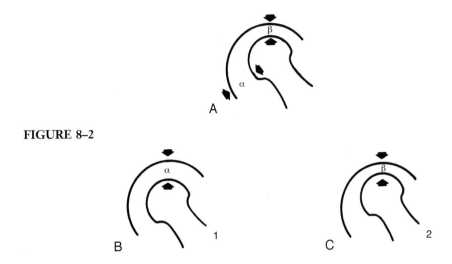

FIGURE 8–2

In a later follow-up study of wear in 547 THJRs using the duoradiographic technique, Griffith and coworkers reported a wear rate of 0.07 mm per year, about half the rate reported by the uniradiographic technique.[7] No reason for this wide discrepancy was offered, despite the facts that the same population of patients was tested, and all the implanted polyethylene cups came from the same source!

"Modern" Techniques of Wear Measurement

Several novel ideas have been introduced to improve the accuracy of radiologic techniques of measuring polyethylene wear. They include an attempt to standardize both the x-rays and the position of the pelvis by the creation of a grid, which ensures reproducible positioning of the hip and the x-ray beam.[8] Another technique measures the distance between the center of the femoral component and that of the acetabular component using a radiograph magnified ten times.[9] All of these improvements in radiologic technique are important, but they can be used only in specialized centers because of their complexity.

The Livermore Technique

In 1990, Livermore and associates published a technique that could be used on plane radiographs in a retrospective manner (Fig. 8–3).[10] It is probably the most commonly used method for long-term radiologic study of acetabular wear. The technique is claimed to have a fivefold increase in accuracy (± 0.1 mm) over previous methods of wear measurement. Despite presenting new data concerning the effect of femoral head size on polyethylene wear, the measurement technique itself was little different from the Charnley duoradiography method, and details of the validation using retrieval implants were not clear. The maximum discrepancy between radiographic and direct measurements of their retrieval implants was 0.4 mm, which is probably a better estimate of the accuracy of the Livermore technique than the 0.1 mm that is claimed. Using this or any other method of linear wear measurement, it is not possible to measure polyethylene wear that occurs in a direction lateral to the opening of the cup. Wroblewski has shown clearly, on the basis of retrieval cups, that it is common for wear to occur in this direction because the head is taking the path of least resistance.[11]

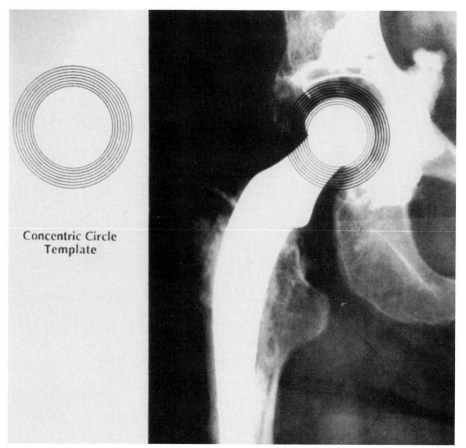

Concentric Circle Template

FIGURE 8-3

Roentgen Stereophotogrammetric Analysis

Roentgen stereophotogrammetric analysis (RSA) is the science of obtaining reliable three-dimensional measurements from radiographs in order to determine primarily the geometric characteristics of an object (Fig. 8–4).[12] Tantalum balls, 0.5 mm or 0.8 mm in diameter, are implanted into the bone at the time of surgery and are later used as radiologic reference markers. RSA has been used for the three-dimensional

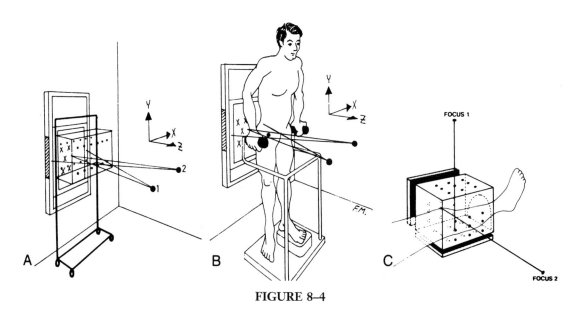

FIGURE 8-4

study of many factors in THJR, including the spatial orientation of the acetabular component,[13] instability,[14] and the measurement of acetabular and femoral anteversion.[15] However, because of its high degree of accuracy, its most important use has been in the assessment of acetabular component migration[16] and polyethylene wear.[17] RSA is the only system used to measure acetabular wear for which accuracy has been fully studied. Comparing RSA and conventional techniques for the measurement of wear suggests that accuracy of RSA is 0.1 mm,[18] whereas the accuracy of conventional techniques is between 0.3 and 0.4 mm.[19]

Maxima Computer Technique

In the late 1980s, a very sophisticated hardware and software was developed to convert radiographs into digital images that could then be analyzed.[20] A combination of interactive and automatic techniques was used to generate a series of reference points on a displayed image of the radiograph. Using an edge-enhancing function on the image, the center of the femoral component and its diameter were found automatically, with great reproducibility ($\pm$ 0.01 mm) (Fig. 8–5). Unfortunately, it is not stated whether the radiographs used were centered on the hip being examined or on the symphysis pubis. In explanation of the relatively poor accuracy of this technique ($\pm$ 0.5 mm) compared to its reproducibility, the comment was made that three-dimensional imaging techniques such as stereophotogrammetry are irrelevant to such a retrospective study for which only plane radiographs are available.[21] The implication was that a major source of error was femoral head displacement out of the plane of the AP radiograph.

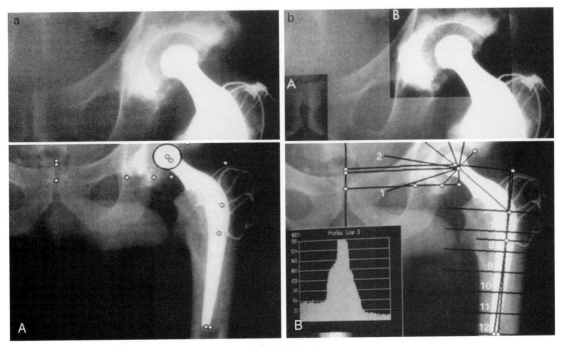

FIGURE 8–5

Three-Dimensional Technique

Dissatisfaction with currently available methodology for measuring polyethylene wear led to the development of the three-dimensional technique.[22] First described in the Frank Stinchfield Award paper at the 1994 open meeting of the Hip Society in New Orleans, it was the first (and so far remains the only) attempt to use information from a shoot-through lateral radiograph (Fig. 8–6). Using information from the radiographic setup, specifically the beam/cassette distance (usually 101.6 cm for the AP radiograph) and the point on the AP radiograph that represents the central beam (Fig. 8–7), points on the periphery of a metal-backed acetabular cup

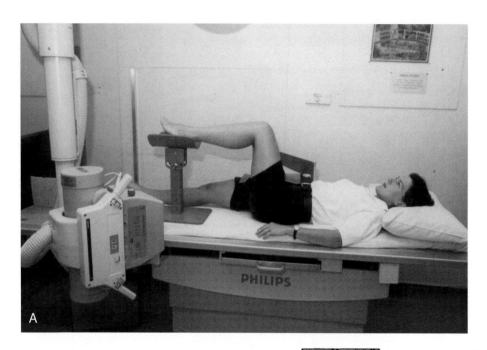

A

FIGURE 8–6

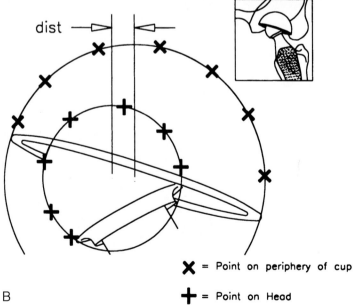

dist

✕ = Point on periphery of cup

+ = Point on Head

B

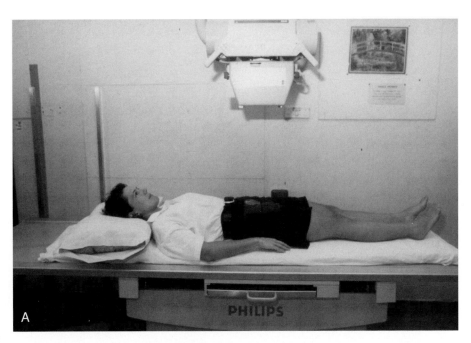

FIGURE 8–7

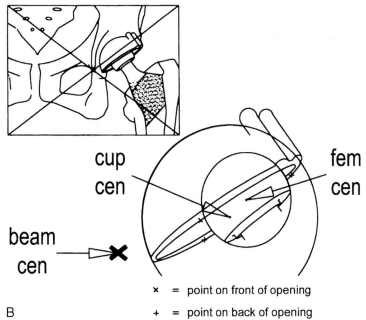

and femoral head are entered into a computer using a back-lit digitizing tablet (Fig. 8–8). Information from the AP and lateral radiograph are combined to build a model of the hip prosthesis in the computer (Fig. 8–9). Correction for different centering of the radiographic beam and variations in pelvic orientation is made by rotating the computer model to a standard frontal view before any measurements of femoral head displacement are made (Fig. 8–10). Comparison of initial postoperative radiographs (assuming no femoral head displacement) and long-term follow-up radiographs (assuming the femoral head lies in the position of maximum wear) allows a calculation of polyethylene wear to be made (assuming the femoral head penetrates into the polyethylene cup in a cylindrical wear pattern).

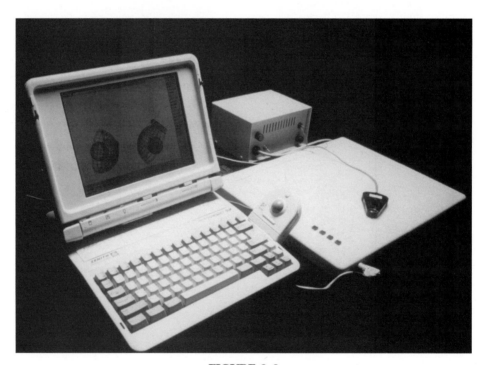

FIGURE 8–8

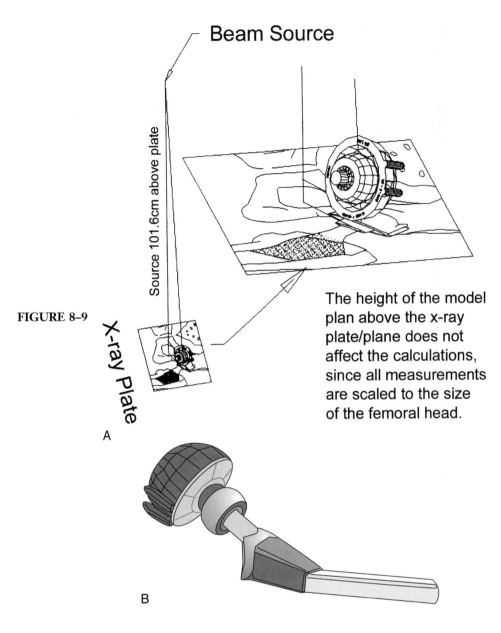

Beam Source

Source 101.6cm above plate

X-ray Plate

FIGURE 8–9

The height of the model plan above the x-ray plate/plane does not affect the calculations, since all measurements are scaled to the size of the femoral head.

A

B

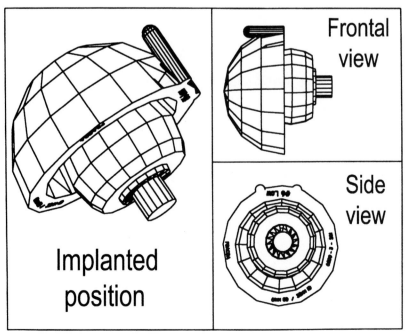

Implanted position

Frontal view

Side view

FIGURE 8–10

145

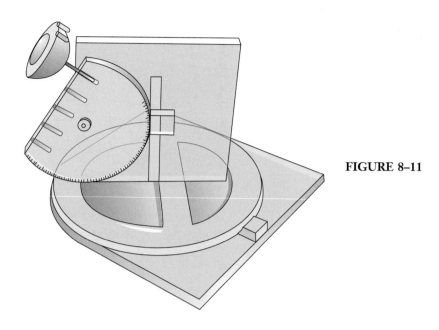

FIGURE 8–11

The accuracy of the three-dimensional technique was assessed by constructing a plexiglass phantom into which a metal-backed acetabular cup could be mounted (Fig. 8–11). Polyethylene wear of the cup was simulated by using a milling machine to remove a precise amount of polyethylene in a known direction (Fig. 8–12). The three-dimensional–technique software was able to predict up to 8.67 mm of femoral head displacement with an accuracy of plus or minus 0.15 mm (Fig. 8–13).[23]

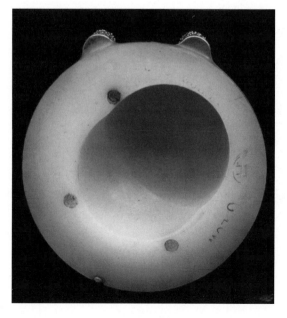

FIGURE 8–12

Accuracy-Wear

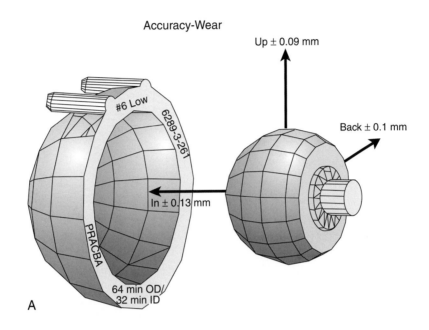

A

FIGURE 8–13

Volume Calculation

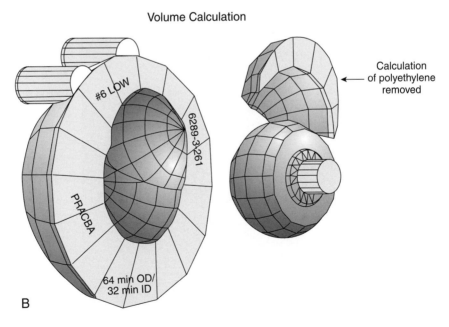

B

Since its initial description as a method requiring AutoCAD (a computer-aided design software package) for implementation, a number of modifications have been made. Not only can it now be applied to an all-polyethylene acetabular cup with a wire marker (Fig. 8–14), it can also use contemporary image processing technology to measure femoral head displacement based on digital images created by scanning radiographs into the computer. These digital images are analyzed using custom filters and edge detectors to generate points from the peripheries of the femoral head and acetabular cup. Although accuracy has been improved only slightly (± 0.09 mm), reproducibility in the form of intra- and interobserver error has been improved fortyfold. This now allows comparison of series from various institutions as well as direct comparison of the polyethylene wear rates of different acetabular cups.

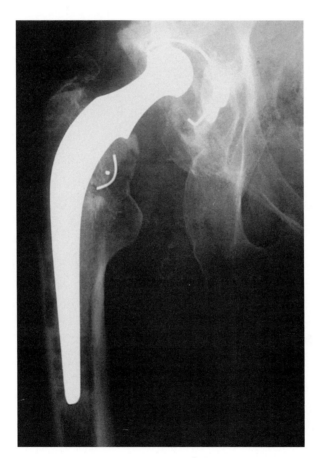

FIGURE 8–14

Digitally Assisted Linear Wear Measurement

Shaver and coworkers have described a method of more accurately analyzing the standardized AP radiograph that provides a highly reproducible measurement of polyethylene wear (Fig. 8–15).[24] It achieves this by digitally locating the margins of the femoral head and acetabular cup using a gradient edge-detector. On the most recent AP radiograph, the shortest distance between the margins is compared to the initial postoperative distance at the same point on the acetabular cup, and the difference is thought to represent polyethylene wear. It is claimed to be accurate enough to predict the long-term wear performance in individual patients by analyzing the measured linear femoral head penetration at 2 years, but this has not yet been proven.

FIGURE 8–15

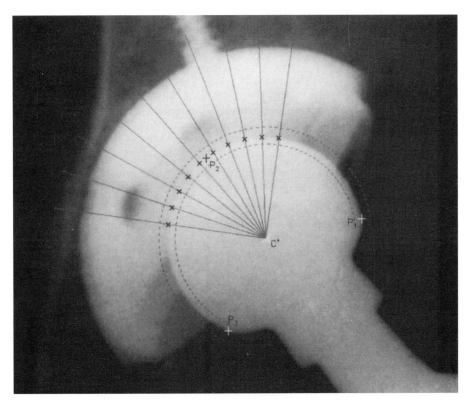

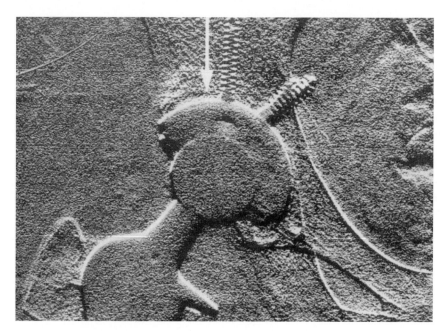

FIGURE 8–16

Martell and Berdia have developed a novel method of linear wear measurement that uses the Hough transform, a computer algorithm for fitting data to known shapes, in this case a circle (Fig. 8–16).[25] Also highly reproducible, this technique has been applied to a series of Harris-Galante prostheses, and retrieval data suggest that this method is also very accurate.

Conclusion

The minimization of polyethylene wear is a major goal of total hip arthroplasty surgeons. Little is known about the factors that influence the rate of wear in a patient. Generation of data from accurate measurement of polyethylene wear may go some way toward addressing these factors. Clinical data generated by measurement methods is only as accurate as the measurement technique itself. Careful validation of all measurement techniques is required, and it must be performed under stringent conditions and peer-reviewed. Much of our early information on polyethylene wear rates has been generated by poor methods and is thus erroneous.

REFERENCES

1. Clarke IC, Black K, Rennie C, et al. Can wear in total hip arthroplasties be assessed from radiographs? Clin Orthop 1976;121:126–142.
2. Charnley J, Kamangar A, Longfield MD. The optimum size of prosthetic heads in relation to the wear of plastic sockets in total replacement of the hip. Med Biol Eng 1969;7:31–39.
3. Walker PS, Salvati EA. The measurement and effects of friction and wear in artificial hip joints. J Biomed Mater Res 1973;7:327–342.
4. Charnley J, Cupic Z. The nine- and ten-year results of the low-friction arthroplasty of the hip. Clin Orthop 1973;95:9–25.
5. Charnley J, Halley DK. Rate of wear in total hip replacement. Clin Orthop 1975;112:170–179.
6. Clarke IC, Gruen TA, Matos M, et al. Improved methods for quantitative radiographic evaluation with particular reference to total-hip arthroplasty. Clin Orthop 1976;121:83–91.
7. Griffith MJ, Seidenstein MK, Williams D, et al. Socket wear in Charnley low-friction arthroplasty of the hip. Clin Orthop 1978;137:37–47.
8. Amstutz HC, Ouzounian T, Grauer D, et al. The grid radiograph: a simple technique for consistent high-resolution visualization of the hip. J Bone Joint Surg 1986;68A:1052–1056.
9. Clarac JP, Pries P, Launay L, et al. Erosion of polyethylene cupulae: radiological study of 123 Charnley total prostheses. Rev Chir Orthop 1986;72:97–100.

10. Livermore J, Ilstrup D, Morrey B. Effect of femoral head size on wear of the polyethylene acetabular component. J Bone Joint Surg 1990;72A:518–528.
11. Wroblewski BM. Direction and rate of socket wear in Charnley low-friction arthroplasty. J Bone Joint Surg 1985;67B:757–761.
12. Selvik G. A roentgen stereophotogrammetric method for study of the kinematics of the skeletal system. Doctor of Philosophy thesis, University of Lund, Sweden, 1974.
13. Herrlin K, Selvik G, Pettersson H. Space orientation of total hip prosthesis: a method for three-dimensional determination. Acta Radiol Diagn Stockh 1986;27:619–627.
14. Baldursson H, Egund N, Hansson LI, et al. Instability and wear of total hip prostheses determined with roentgen stereophotogrammetry. Arch Orthop Trauma Surg 1979;95:257–263.
15. Wientroub S, Boyde A, Chrispin AR, et al. The use of stereophotogrammetry to measure acetabular and femoral anteversion. J Bone Joint Surg 1981;63B:209–213.
16. Baldursson H, Hansson LI, Olsson TH, et al. Migration of the acetabular socket after total hip replacement determined by roentgen stereophotogrammetry. Acta Orthop Scand 1980;51:535–540.
17. Franzen H, Mjoberg B. Wear and loosening of the hip prosthesis: a roentgen stereophotogrammetric 3-year study of 14 cases. Acta Orthop Scand 1990;61:499–501.
18. Selvik G, Alberius P, Aronson AS. A roentgen stereophotogrammetric system: construction, calibration and technical accuracy. Acta Radiol Diagn Stockh 1983;24:343–352.
19. Ilchmann T. Radiographic assessment of cup migration and wear after hip replacement. Acta Orthop Scand Suppl 1997;276:1–26.
20. Jones PR, Taylor CJ, Hukins DW, et al. Prosthetic hip failure: retrospective radiograph image analysis of the acetabular cup. J Biomed Eng 1989;11:253–257.
21. Jones PR, Taylor CJ, Hukins DW, et al. Prosthetic hip failure: preliminary findings of retrospective radiograph image analysis. Eng Med 1988;17:119–125.
22. Devane PA. The measurement of polyethylene wear in metal-backed acetabular components. Master of Science thesis, University of Western Ontario, London, Ontario, Canada, 1993.
23. Devane PA, Bourne RB, Rorabeck CH, et al. Measurement of polyethylene wear in metal-backed acetabular cups. I. Three-dimensional technique. Clin Orthop 1995;319:303–316.
24. Shaver SM, Brown TD, Hillis SL, et al. Digital edge-detection measurement of polyethylene wear after total hip arthroplasty. J Bone Joint Surg 1997;79A:690–700.
25. Martell JM, Berdia S. Determination of polyethylene wear in total hip replacements with use of digital radiographs. J Bone Joint Surg 1997;79A:1635–1641.

9

Hydroxyapatite-Coated Femoral Components

DANIEL J. BERRY

BRIAN J. McGRORY

Hydroxyapatite is a bioactive calcium phosphate ceramic material that can be applied in a thin layer to metallic prosthetic implants.[1] Hydroxyapatite is osteoconductive; bone can form in direct apposition to hydroxyapatite, and such bone ongrowth can provide stable biologic fixation of orthopedic implants.[1]

Hydroxyapatite has been applied to smooth, textured, and rough metal surfaces and to both acetabular and femoral components. In general, more reliable bone ongrowth and more stable implant fixation has been reported with hydroxyapatite-coated femoral components than with acetabular components.

Radiographic characteristics of well-fixed hydroxyapatite-coated sockets include (1) a stable implant without migration or change in position and (2) no new radiolucent lines at the bone/implant interface. Signs suggestive of loosening include change in implant position or inclination and formation of a new radiolucent line at the bone/prosthesis interface. An early finding suggestive of loosening is a new radiolucent line at the bone/implant interface of the inferior medial aspect of the socket. This is indicative of early vertical tilting of the socket.

On the femoral side, radiographic changes around hydroxyapatite-coated implants are more profound because bone remodeling around well-fixed components is more readily visible. Many implants are only partially coated with hydroxyapatite, and parallel radiolucent or radiodense lines around the implant in those areas are common (Figs. 9–1 through 9–3).[2-5] Well-fixed implants typically show no radiolucent line at the prosthesis-bone interface in the areas in which the implant is coated (Figs. 9–2 through 9–5). Thus, knowing which regions of a particular implant are coated with hydroxyapatite is essential for accurate interpretation of the radiographs.

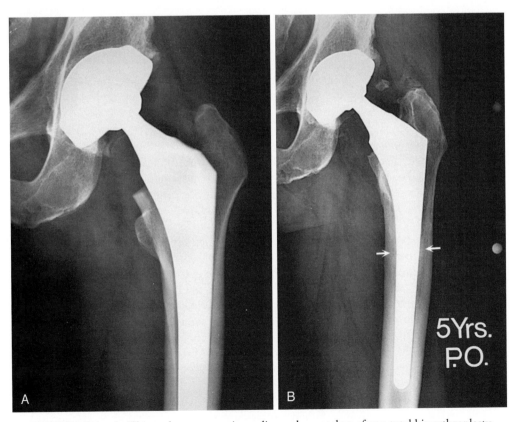

FIGURE 9–1 **A:** This early postoperative radiograph was taken after a total hip arthroplasty that employed a hydroxyapatite-coated femoral component. **B:** This radiograph was taken 5 years after the total hip arthroplasty. The implant is stable. There are no radiolucent lines around the proximal stem where hydroxyapatite coating is present. Condensation of cancellous bone around the hydroxyapatite-coated portion of the stem is visible, particularly at the distal extent of the coating (arrows). The parallel radiolucent and radiodense lines around the distal, uncoated portion of the stem do not indicate loosening. There is mild bone atrophy of the femoral neck consistent with stress shielding.

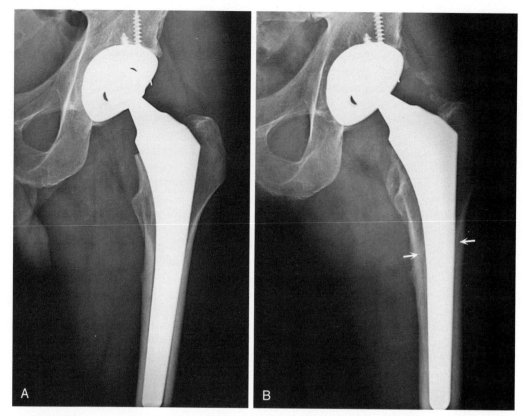

FIGURE 9–2   A: This early postoperative radiograph was taken after a total hip arthroplasty involving a hydroxyapatite-coated femoral component. **B:** A radiograph taken 4 years later demonstrates the typical radiographic findings of a well-fixed femoral component proximally coated with hydroxyapatite. Cortical hypertrophy and cancellous bone condensation may be seen around the midportion of the implant, that is, the distal extent of the hydroxyapatite coating (arrows).

With time, usually 1 to 2 years after implantation, bone remodeling becomes radiographically visible around hydroxyapatite femoral components that have become osteointegrated. The earliest findings typically are condensations of cancellous bone near the most distal aspects of the hydroxyapatite coating (see Figs. 9–1 through 9–3).[2-5] With time, there may also be hypertrophy of the cortical bone in these regions (see Figs. 9–2 and 9–3).[2-5] If the implant is coated only proximally with hydroxyapatite, it is typical to see condensations at the metaphyseal/diaphyseal junction. Eventually, cortical condensation may occur around much of the implant. Proximal bone atrophy, particularly of the femoral neck, is common around well-fixed femoral implants and is indicative of stress shielding (see Fig. 9–1).

Loose hydroxyapatite-coated femoral implants typically demonstrate migration or subsidence of the implant relative to fixed femoral landmarks (see Fig. 9–5). A complete radiolucent line at the prosthesis/bone interface may also be seen (see Fig. 9–5). Nonparallel radiolucent lines around the stem are usually indicative of implant motion and loosening.

Pedestal formation and cortical hypertrophy can occur near the tip of both well-fixed and loose implants. When associated with loose femoral implants, cortical hypertrophy and pedestal formation is thought to occur as the result of a bony reaction related to the implant's motion. Thus, the significance of cortical hypertrophy near the tip of the implant must be considered in the context of other radiographic findings.

Radiographic changes around hydroxyapatite-coated implants used for femoral component revision surgery are similar to those described after primary total hip arthroplasty (see Fig. 9–5). Revision femoral components are often longer and may

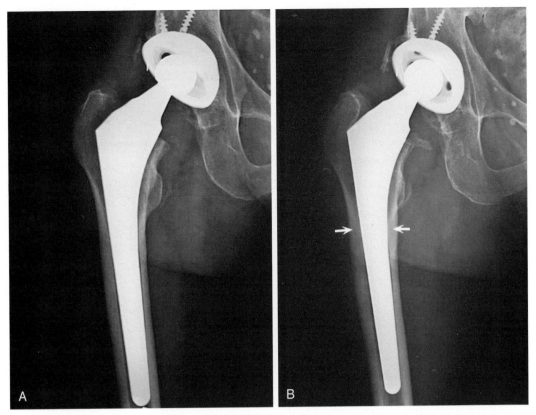

FIGURE 9–3   A: This early postoperative radiograph was taken after a total hip arthroplasty employing a hydroxyapatite-coated femoral component. **B:** A radiograph taken 4 years later demonstrates the typical findings of a well-fixed femoral component coated with hydroxyapatite. Cancellous bone condensation and cortical hypertrophy may be noted at the distant extent of the hydroxyapatite coating (arrows).

FIGURE 9–4   A: This early postoperative radiograph was taken after a total hip arthroplasty that employed a hydroxyapatite-coated femoral component. **B:** In a radiograph taken 1 year later, the femoral component is loose. Subsidence and a tilt to the varus position may be seen, along with radiolucent lines around the stem, including the superior part of the stem that is hydroxyapatite-coated.

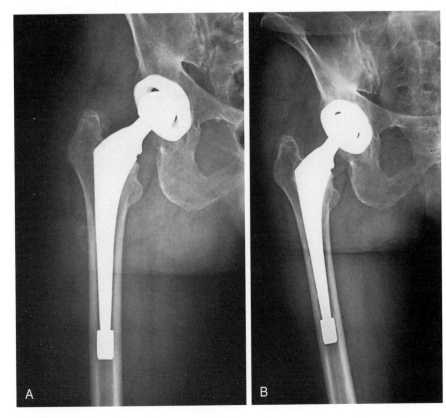

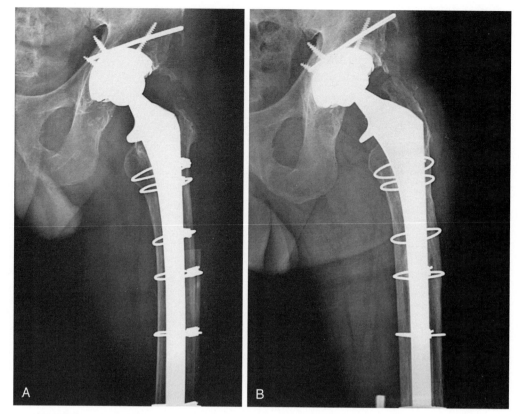

FIGURE 9–5 A: This early postoperative radiograph was taken after revision total hip arthroplasty that involved a hydroxyapatite-coated stem and cortical strut bone allografts. **B:** This radiograph was taken 5 years later. The stem is well fixed. There is cancellous bone condensation at the distal border of the coating, and parallel radiodense lines are present around the distal uncoated stem.

have hydroxyapatite coating that extends more distally on the stem; bone remodeling reflects these differences (see Fig. 9–5).

REFERENCES

1. Geesink RGT, Manley MT. Hydroxyapatite Coatings in Orthopaedic Surgery. New York, Raven Press, 1993.
2. D'Antonio JA, Capello WN, Crothers OD, et al. Early clinical experience with hydroxyapatite-coated implants. J Bone Joint Surg 1992;74A:995–1008.
3. Geesink RGT, Hoefnagels NHM. Hydroxyapatite coatings: clinical and retrieval analysis data. In Sedel L, Cabanela ME, eds. Hip Surgery: Materials and Developments. London, Martin Dunitz, 1998, pp. 253–265.
4. Geesink RGT, Hoefnagels NHM. Six-year results of hydroxyapatite-coated total hip replacement. J Bone Joint Surg 1995;77B:534–547.
5. Geesink RGT. Hydroxyapatite-coated total hip replacement, two-year clinical and radiological results. Clin Orthop 1990;261:39–58.

10

—

Primary and Revision Arthroplasty of the Knee

—

DAVID C. MARKEL

Total knee arthroplasty has developed rapidly since its introduction in the early 1970s. Implant designs and surgical techniques have gone through significant evolution during this time. Some of the important developments include refinements in metallurgy, improved polymers and polyethylene, an understanding of metal and plastic biomechanics, universal instrumentation, and ligament balancing. There are still fundamental differences in opinion regarding component design, the status of the posterior cruciate ligament, the need to resurface the patella, and the use of cement. Despite these differences, the art and science of knee arthroplasty have reached a point where one can expect accurate limb alignment and excellent long-term results with nearly all the current implant systems.

Total knee arthroplasty has rapidly become the gold standard for treatment of arthritis of the knee. This is due in part to the success of the procedure. In appropriately selected patients, good to excellent results are to be expected in 95% of patients, and the survival rate of the knee is expected to be 95% at 15 years. Future implant designs may prove to be even more successful than those used in the past.

Despite the broad success of total knee arthroplasty, complications and problems do arise. Most of them can be diagnosed clinically or radiographically. The examples provided here highlight successful and failed reconstructions of straightforward and complex knee pathology (Figs. 10–1 through 10–29).

Text continued on page 181

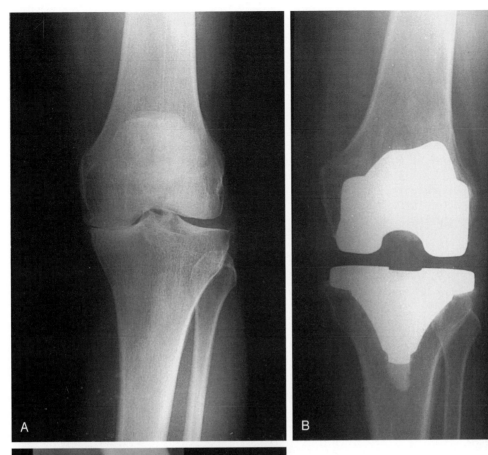

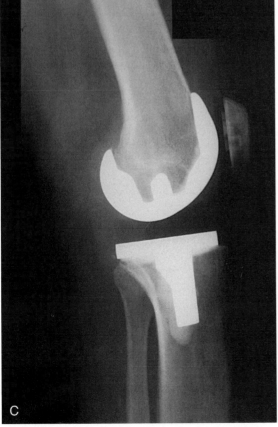

FIGURE 10–1 A: Preoperative anteroposterior (AP) radiograph of a knee with varus arthritis and obliteration of the medial compartment with weight-bearing. **B** and **C:** Postoperative AP and lateral radiographs of an uncomplicated knee replacement. The femoral component's metal contour matches that of the bone, there is good bony coverage, the patella is at an appropriate height, and there is a mild anatomic posterior tibial slope. The limb alignment has been restored to slight valgus.

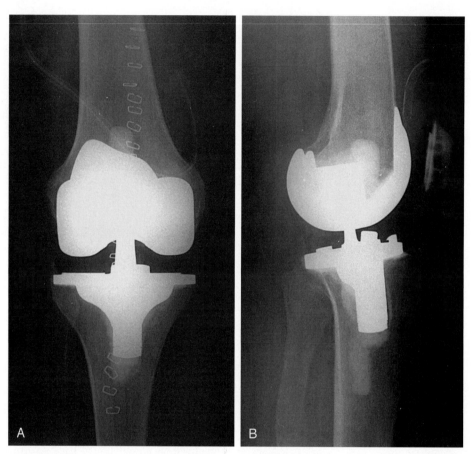

FIGURE 10–2 A and **B:** AP and lateral radiographs of a posterior stabilized cruciate-sacrificing knee component. A polyethylene post extends from the tibial tray and is housed in the metallic box shown on the lateral film. The plastic post and the metallic housing interact to provide increased stability and substitute for the cruciate ligament. Surgical staples are in the skin for wound closure. A drain is noted within the joint to evacuate any hematomas.

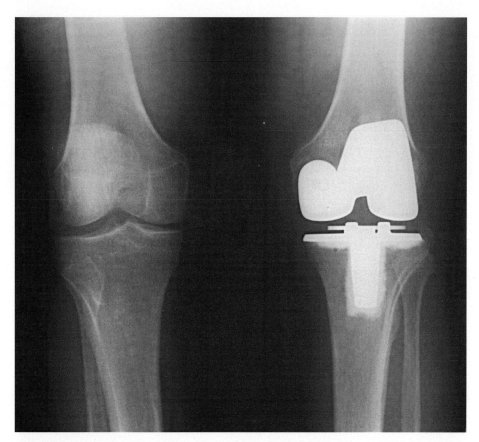

FIGURE 10–3 AP radiograph of a cemented cruciate-sacrificing knee design. The polyeth-ylene is locked into the tibial tray with the crosspin-like mechanism. Slight external rotation of the femoral component is evident; the posterior medial flange is more prominent, whereas the tibial component appears true.

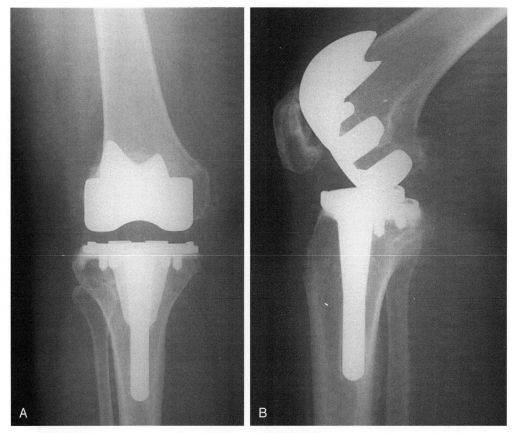

FIGURE 10–4 **A** and **B:** AP and lateral radiographs of a hybrid knee replacement. The femoral component is uncemented; the patella and tibial components are cemented.

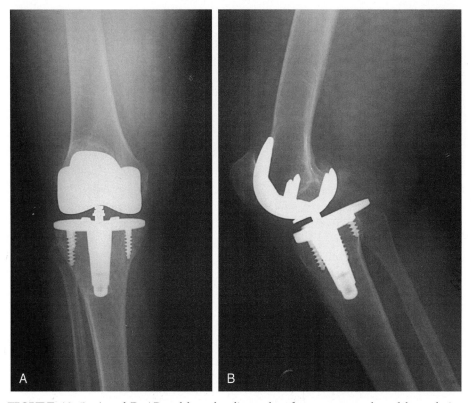

FIGURE 10–5 **A** and **B:** AP and lateral radiographs of an uncemented total knee design. The screws are intended to provide initial stability during the period of ingrowth. Osteolysis is noted at the distal ends of the screws as a result of polyethylene wear. Rarefaction of the distal femur is the result of stress shielding.

FIGURE 10–6   A and **B:** AP and lateral radiographs of a well-fit and well-positioned, cemented, semiconstrained, stemmed total knee arthroplasty. The femoral component appears to be appropriately sized, and it matches the contours of the bone. The tibial component has good coverage of the bone, and the stems are central in the canals and do not translate the components. The metallic box seen on the lateral film houses a post to provide increased stability and constraint in the mediolateral plane.

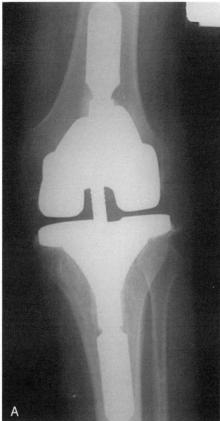
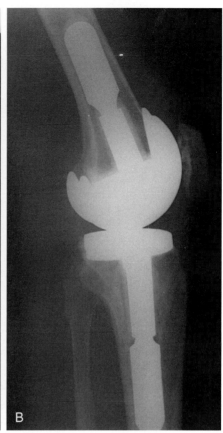

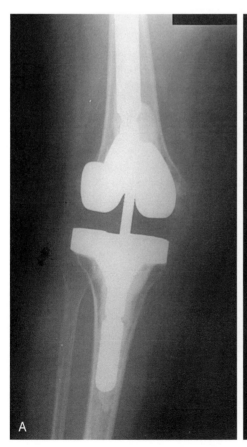
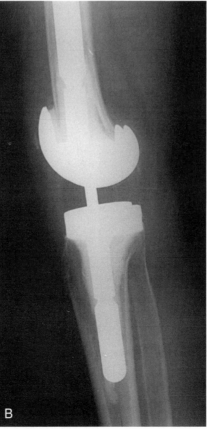

FIGURE 10–7   A and **B:** AP and lateral postoperative radiographs of a rheumatoid patient who underwent revision to a semiconstrained style of knee design. The tibial component was thickened with metallic augments, and a thick polyethylene insert was used to achieve ligamentous stability and to correct for bone loss. Stems were used to provide biomechanical advantage because constraint and augments were applied. The metal rod seen between the components reinforces a plastic post that fits tightly into the femoral component and provides mediolateral stability.

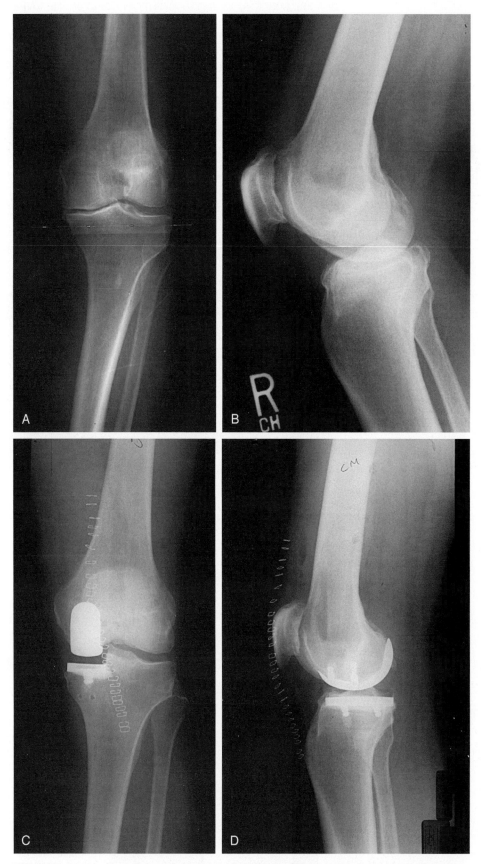

FIGURE 10–8 A and **B:** AP and lateral radiographs of a knee demonstrating varus gonarthrosis. The lateral compartment and the patellofemoral joint appear to be relatively well preserved. **C** and **D:** AP and lateral radiographs after unicondylar knee arthroplasty. The limb alignment appears to have been restored to a slight valgus inclination, and the arthritis in the medial joint compartment has been addressed.

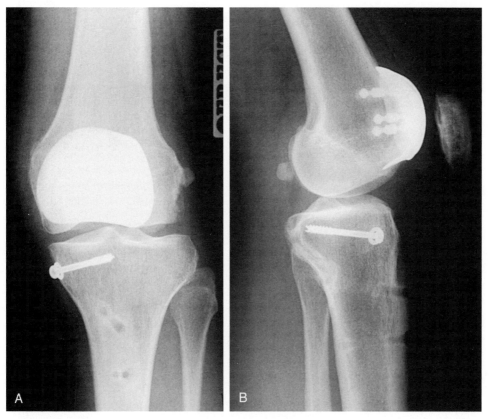

FIGURE 10–9 A and **B:** AP and lateral radiographs of another form of unicompartmental arthroplasty. This patellofemoral replacement resurfaces the trochlea with metal and the patella with plastic. These implants are not widely used, although new designs are being investigated. The tibial screw and drill holes are remnants of unrelated trauma.

FIGURE 10–10 AP radiographs of bilateral total knee replacements. One knee appears to be well-aligned and well-positioned. The other knee appears to be incompletely seated on the lateral side; it is likely that the soft medial cancellous bone collapsed during cement pressurization. The projection shows the knee in a flexed posture, which represents a potential flexion contracture.

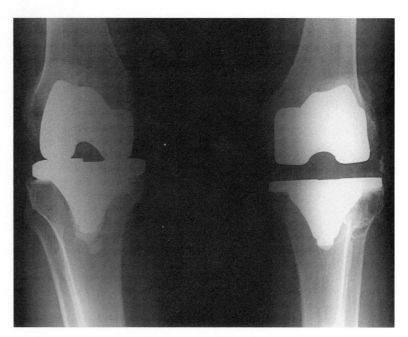

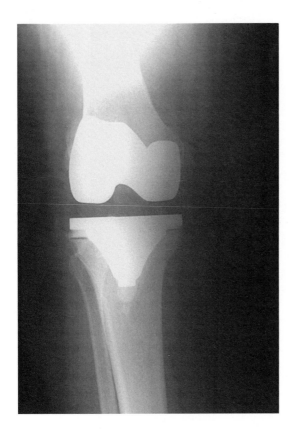

FIGURE 10–11 AP radiograph of a standard total knee replacement. The tibial component was incompletely seated during cementing.

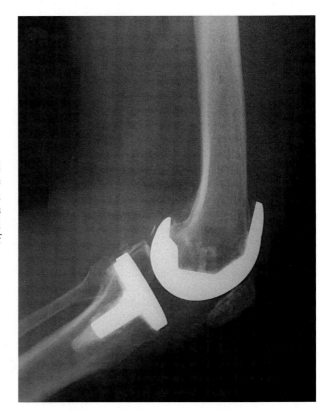

FIGURE 10–12 Lateral radiograph of a cemented total knee arthroplasty. A thin layer of cement is evident on the posterior aspect of the polyethylene. The cement is not on the articulating surface and should not be a problem unless it breaks free. In addition, it appears that a generous distal femoral resection was made, causing proximal overhang of the femoral component.

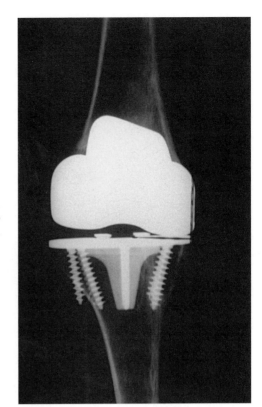

FIGURE 10–13 AP radiograph of an uncemented knee replacement. The polyethylene on the medial side is severely worn, causing the knee to fall into varus. Osteolysis is evident, particularly next to the medial screws.

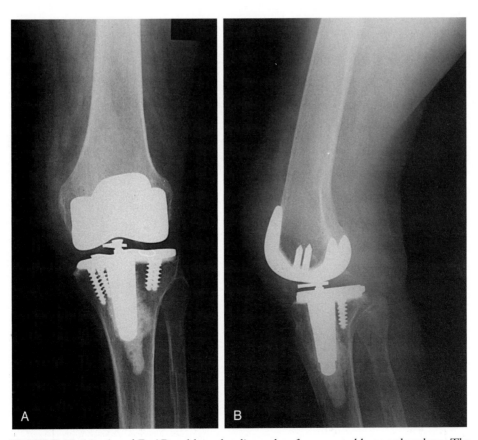

FIGURE 10–14 **A** and **B:** AP and lateral radiographs of a cemented knee arthroplasty. The knee was unstable. Posterior sag of the tibial component is evident on the lateral film. Metallic wear is evident on the medial side of the tibial tray (the corner is rounded off).

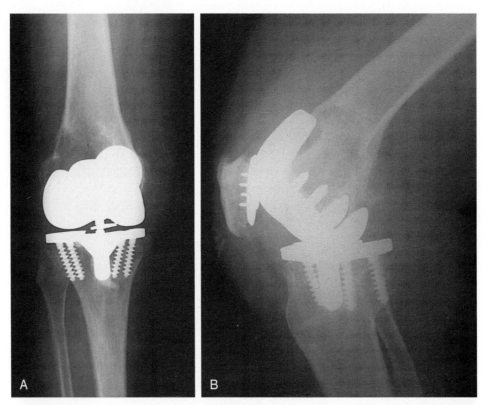

FIGURE 10–15   AP and lateral radiographs of a hybrid total knee arthroplasty (cemented tibia, uncemented femoral component). The patella is uncemented and metal-backed. **A:** On the AP film, a large osteolytic lesion is noted in the distal lateral femur. Lesions are also noted in the proximal tibia. **B:** The lateral radiograph reveals that the osteolysis and bone loss involve the entire AP dimension of the femur.

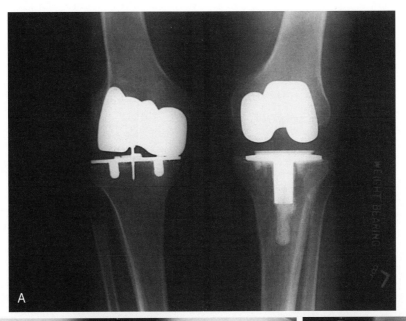

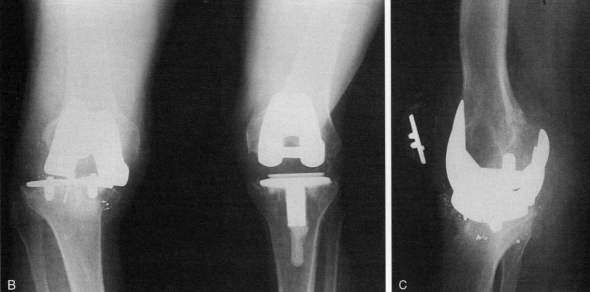

FIGURE 10–16 **A:** AP radiograph of bilateral knee arthroplasties, one cemented, one uncemented. The uncemented knee has severe polyethylene wear that causes the component to be unstable and fall into varus. Metallic wear should also be suspected. The opposite knee is stable, well fixed, and has thick polyethylene. **B** and **C:** AP and lateral radiographs of the same patient 1 year later. The wear and loosening have progressed. The tibial component has fractured. Large osteolytic lesions are noted in the femur and in the anterior tibia on the lateral film. The knee is grossly unstable upon examination and exhibits tibial femoral subluxation on the AP film. The opposite knee was imaged in a flexed position.

Illustration continued on following page

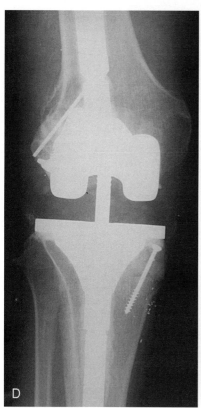

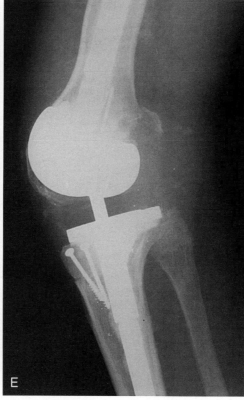

FIGURE 10–16 *Continued.* **D** and **E:** AP and lateral radiographs of the revision arthroplasty. Allograft bone was applied to the anterior and medial aspect of the tibia as well as to the lateral femoral condyle. The allograft was fixed with interfragmentary screws and pins. Long-stemmed components and a metallic posterolateral femoral augment were applied to help provide increased structural stability to the construct.

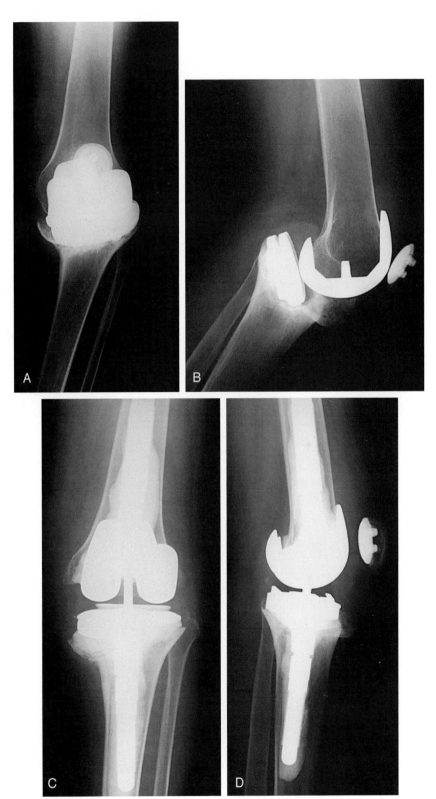

FIGURE 10–17   A and **B:** AP and lateral radiographs of a failed uncemented knee arthroplasty. The femur appears to be well fixed and stable, but there is significant rarefaction of the bone in the anterior part of the femur. The tibia has collapsed, the medial cortex has fractured, and there is significant bone loss. **C** and **D:** AP and lateral radiographs after revision to a cemented, stemmed, semiconstrained component. The modular stems were cemented over their entire length. The metal-backed patella was well fixed and was not revised.

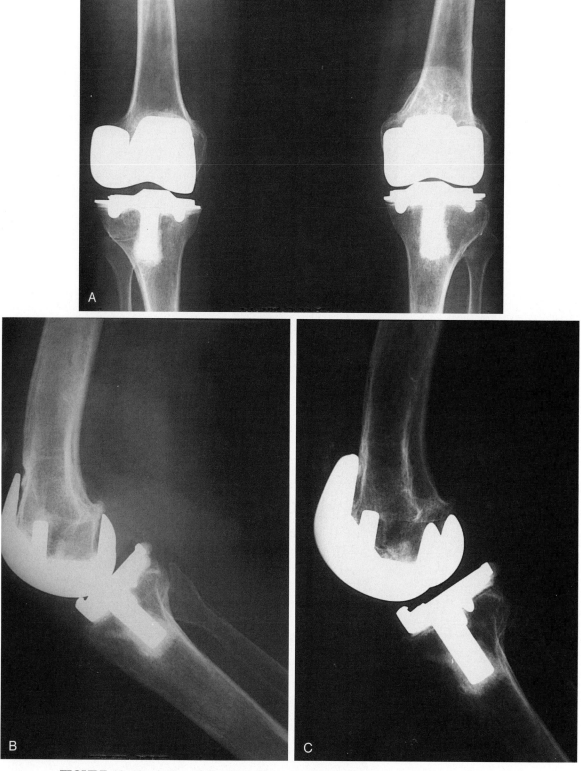

FIGURE 10–18 A, B, and **C:** AP and lateral radiographs of an aging knee implant. Areas of bone resorption may be noted anteriorly and posteriorly. The anterior femoral cortices were notched at the index procedure. Loosening may be noted beneath the tibial tray.

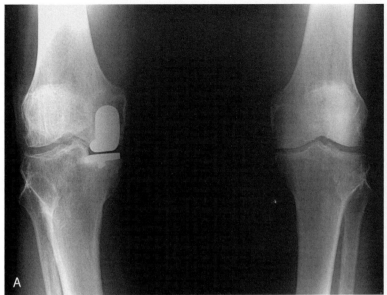

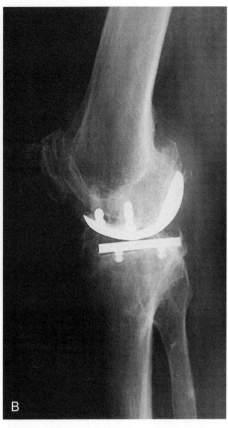

FIGURE 10–19 **A** and **B:** AP and lateral radiographs of a unicondylar knee replacement. The implant initially provided relief, but arthritis in the patellofemoral and lateral compartments became disabling. The generous tibial resection level should be noted as part of the preoperative plan for revision surgery.

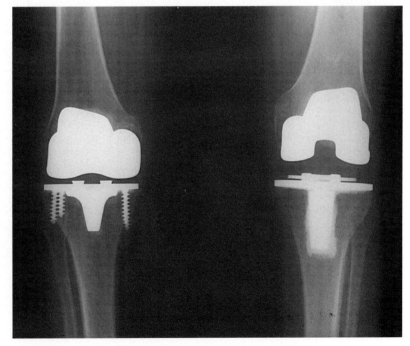

FIGURE 10–20 AP radiograph of bilateral knee arthroplasties. The right knee is uncemented. The prominent anteromedial screw caused pes anserine bursitis. The left knee has thick polyethylene. The thick component was added during a revision arthroplasty for symptoms of instability.

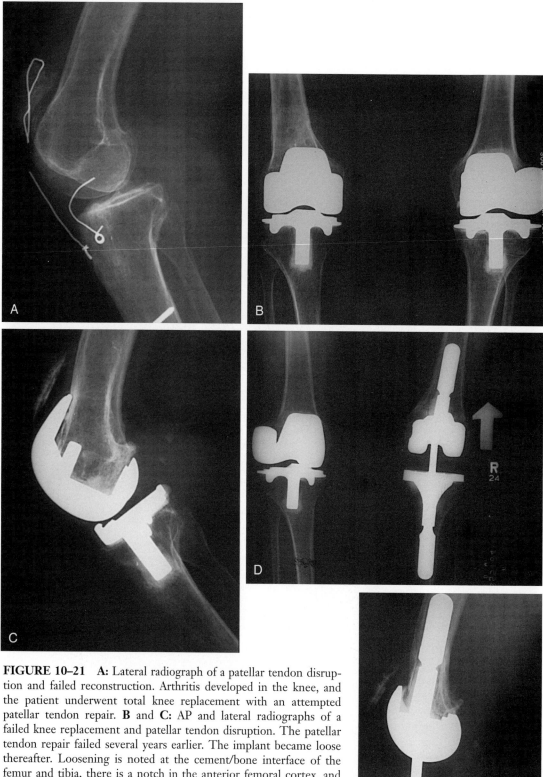

FIGURE 10–21   A: Lateral radiograph of a patellar tendon disruption and failed reconstruction. Arthritis developed in the knee, and the patient underwent total knee replacement with an attempted patellar tendon repair. **B** and **C:** AP and lateral radiographs of a failed knee replacement and patellar tendon disruption. The patellar tendon repair failed several years earlier. The implant became loose thereafter. Loosening is noted at the cement/bone interface of the femur and tibia, there is a notch in the anterior femoral cortex, and the patella is in a significantly proximal (alta) position. **D** and **E:** Postoperative AP and lateral radiographs of the reconstruction. Semitendinosus and gracilis grafts were harvested and used to restrain the patella. Stemmed, semiconstrained components were cemented in place, and a metallic augment was used on the medial tibia to correct for bone loss. A very thick polyethylene insert was required to stabilize the attenuated collateral ligaments. Although the patella is still a bit high, the patient has active extension and no significant extensor lag. The opposite knee is in slight varus, and somewhat unstable, but has not yet caused problems for the patient.

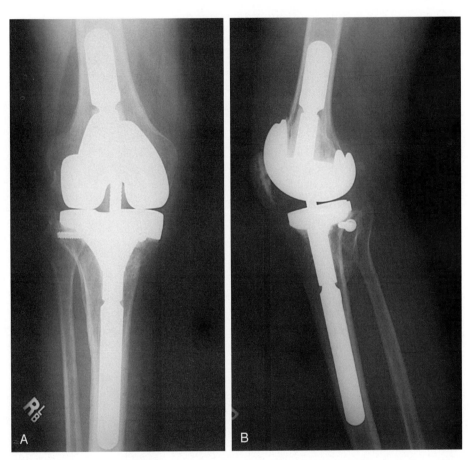

FIGURE 10–22   **A** and **B:** AP and lateral radiographs of a cemented, stemmed, semicon-strained knee replacement. The patient had posttraumatic arthritis after a severe proximal tibial fracture. At the time of surgery, a tibial nonunion was reduced with an interfragmentary screw. A metallic wedge was used to augment the medial aspect of the tibial component and to correct for bone loss.

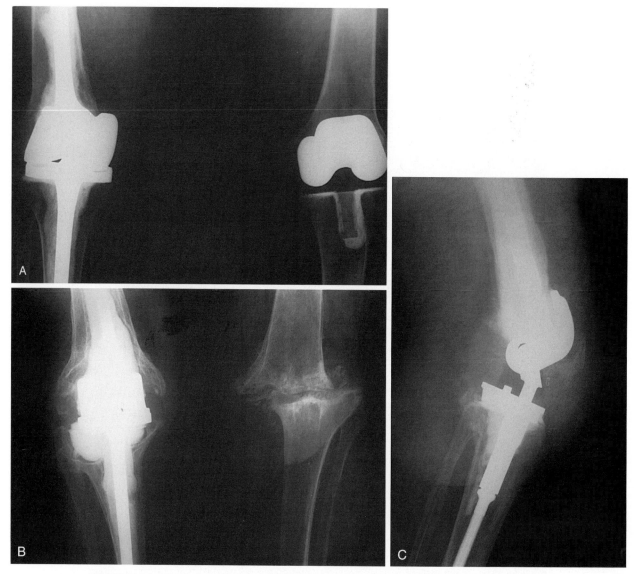

FIGURE 10–23   A: AP radiograph of bilateral knee arthroplasties. Both knees are cemented. One knee is a more conventional condylar knee with an all-polyethylene tibial component. The other knee is a stemmed, constrained knee (a linked-hinge). There does not appear to be much joint space due to wear of the polyethylene inserts. **B:** AP radiograph of the same knees after resection arthroplasty performed because of infection. The constrained knee has continued to wear and loosen. Significant bone loss is evident in the distal femur and proximal tibia. **C:** Lateral radiograph of the revision surgery. Conversion to a modern constrained, hinged knee was performed. The femoral and tibial components are linked through the metal post at the posterior femoral condyle.

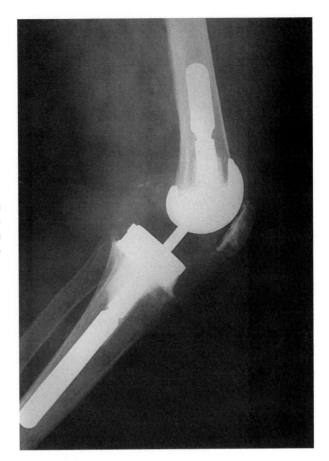

FIGURE 10–24   Lateral radiograph of a revision total knee arthroplasty. Metallic tibial augments and a thick polyethylene insert were used to correct for bone loss. The joint line was raised during the reconstruction, resulting in a patella infera.

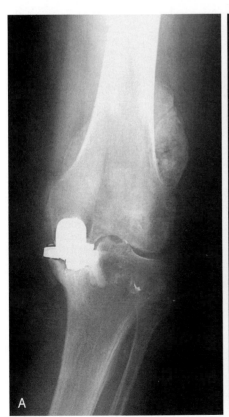

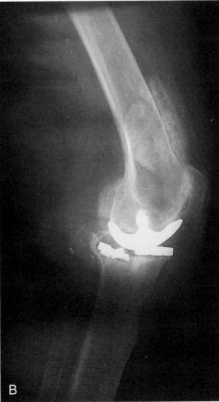

FIGURE 10–25 A and **B:** AP and lateral radiographs of a loose, failed unicondylar knee. The loose component has fractured on the tibial side, causing increased bone loss. Arthritis is evident in the other two compartments, and heterotopic bone is present in the suprapatellar pouch.

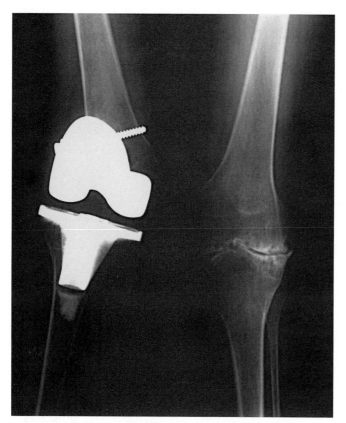

FIGURE 10–26   AP radiograph of a patient with juvenile rheumatoid arthritis. An intraoperative fracture occurred through the femoral condyle. The fracture was fixed with an interfragmentary screw. Poor bone stock and poor patient compliance led to the failure and collapse of the construct. The fracture healed in a significantly valgus position. The knee was not painful, but the patient was very unhappy with the angled extremity and the increasing pain in her arthritic hip. The opposite knee has significant valgus arthritis.

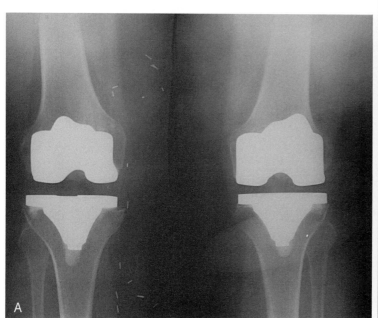
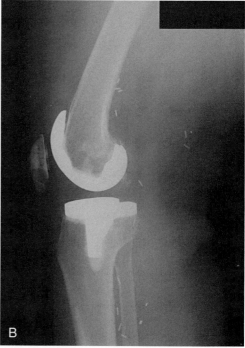

FIGURE 10–27   **A** and **B:** AP and lateral radiographs of cemented knee arthroplasties. The tibial component on the right knee is slightly undersized and lateralized on the AP film. On the lateral film, slight flexion of the femoral component is evident. More importantly, a fracture is noted at the distal pole of the patella. The fracture occurred 1 year after surgery. The fragment was minimally displaced, and the patellar component was not compromised. The fracture healed uneventfully.

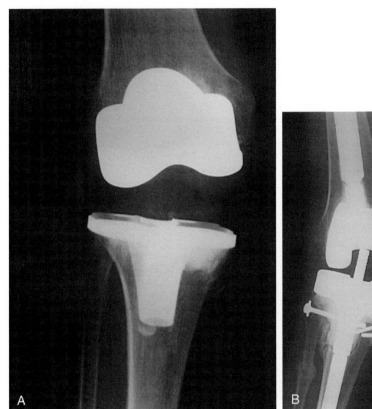

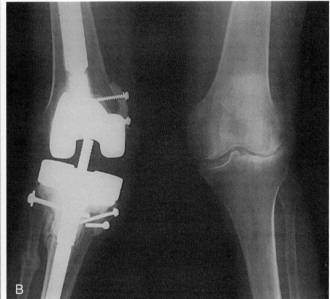

FIGURE 10–28 A: AP radiograph of a failed cruciate-retaining knee arthroplasty. The medial collateral ligament was compromised at surgery and not corrected. The patient had a valgus thrust and medial opening of the knee during weightbearing (this is not a stress view). **B:** AP radiograph of the revision arthroplasty of the knee. A thick polyethylene insert and tibial augments were used to tighten the ligamentous complexes. A medial collateral ligament reconstruction was attempted with a patellar/tendon allograft. The allograft failed after 5 months. The constraining post proved ineffective, and the knee remained unstable.

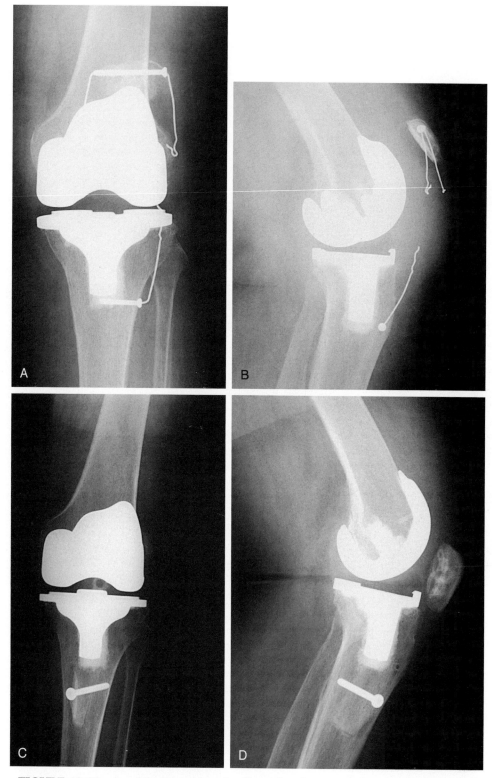

FIGURE 10–29 **A** and **B:** AP and lateral radiographs of a cemented knee arthroplasty after patellar tendon disruption and failed repair. The wires were previously linked in attempt to protect the repair during healing. The repair failed, resulting in patella alta. **C** and **D:** AP and lateral radiographs of the knee after allograft reconstruction of the extensor mechanism. Distally, the tibial screw secures the allograft bone block to the host. The allograft quadriceps tendon was sewn into the host proximally. A patellar button was cemented into the allograft patella. The repaired patella is in a significantly distal (baha) position.

BIBLIOGRAPHY

Dumbleton JH. Wear and prosthetic joints. In Morrey BF, Reconstructive Surgery of the Joints, 2nd ed. New York: Churchill Livingstone, 1996, pp. 61–73.

Insall JN, Salvati EA. Patella position in the normal knee joint. Radiology 1971;101:101–104.

Lotke P. Surgical reconstruction of the arthritic knee. Orthop Clin North Am 1989;20:1.

Lowry Barnes C, Barrach R, Dennis D, et al. Knee reconstruction. In Beaty JH, ed. Rosemont, IL: AAOS, 1999, pp. 559–582.

Morrey BF. Reconstructive Surgery of the Joints, 2nd ed. New York: Churchill Livingstone, 1996, pp. 1345–1586. Rand J, section editor.

Windsor RE, Insall JN, Sculco TP. Bone grafting of tibial defects in primary and revision total knee arthroplasty. Clin Orthop 1986;205:132–137.

11

Ultrasound of Joint Replacements

RONALD S. ADLER

The utility of ultrasound in the evaluation of joint prostheses arises from its excellent depiction of the periprosthetic soft tissues without image distortion in the presence of the indwelling metallic hardware. Indeed, metal and polyethylene present their own characteristic appearances on ultrasound. As a result, bone/metal and metal/polyethylene interfaces can be evaluated, provided there is adequate acoustic access. The presence of periprosthetic fluid, soft-tissue masses, and joint effusions is well depicted by ultrasound. Because it occurs in real time and is steriotactic, ultrasound can provide localization and continuous monitoring of needle placement during aspirations. Further, capsular and synovial biopsies as well as biopsies of soft-tissue masses are easily performed under ultrasound guidance. In view of these favorable properties, it is surprising that there is a relative paucity in the medical literature of reports about the use of ultrasound in patients with indwelling prostheses. Several papers have illustrated the potential of evaluating periprosthetic fluid collections and polyethylene wear.[1, 2]

This chapter illustrates these applications as well as several other circumstances in which ultrasound is expected to be useful in this population of patients. These applications of ultrasound are illustrated by images combined with detailed descriptions. The ultrasound appearances of a total knee replacement are described and attention is given to polyethylene wear and associated wear-debris synovitis. The appearance of joint fluid and periprosthetic fluid collections is discussed with regard to hip replacements. It should be noted that the principles illustrated are the same regardless of anatomic location and type of prosthesis imaged. Ultrasound images obtained in patients without joint replacements are used in several examples to illustrate specific points that are relevant to the theme of this chapter (Figs. 11–1 through 11–14).

Text continued on page 196

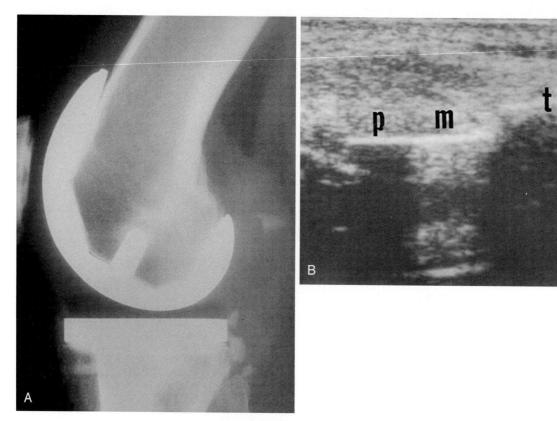

FIGURE 11–1   A: This lateral radiograph of the knee shows a newly placed nonconstrained total knee prosthesis with patellar resurfacing. The lucent zone situated between the metallic tibial tray and the femoral component represents the polyethylene spacer. **B:** This longitudinal sonogram was obtained over the anterior aspect of the lateral compartment in the same patient. The horizontally oriented echogenic (bright) line on the right denotes the cortical surface of the tibial metaphysis (t). The lack of sound transmission beyond the cortical surface manifests as an acoustic shadow (dark zone). Echoes (bright spots) that appear below this boundary are caused by repeated reflections from the transducer surface and are referred to as reverberations. To the left of this cortical margin, a transition occurs to a second horizontally oriented line. The shadow beyond the line first appears bright (echogenic) and then dark (hypoechoic). The first zone is the characteristic acoustic signature of a metallic interface (m) (a tibial tray in this case); the second component is the polyethylene spacer (p). This shadow/ echo/shadow complex depicts the bone/metal/polyethylene surfaces.

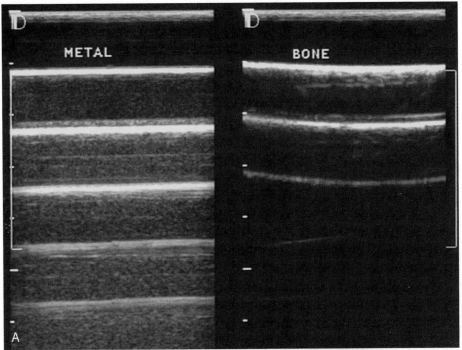

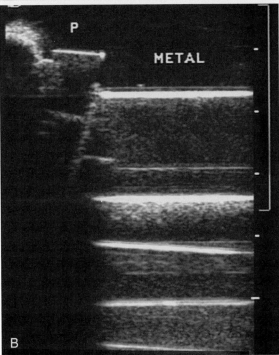

FIGURE 11–2 These are the ultrasound images of bone, metal, and polyethylene immersed in a water bath. **A:** A split ultrasound image was taken of a bone specimen from the femur of a cow (right) and a metallic aluminum block (left) using identical ultrasound parameters. Both materials are strong reflectors of ultrasound and result in multiple linear reverberations below the principal reflection (immediately below label). Metal is characteristically distinguished by the presence of extensive noise (white speckles) and contains many more reverberations than the bone interface. **B:** These are the images of a polyethylene spacer and an aluminum block using the same settings used in part A. The letter P denotes the polyethylene (left). Polyethylene also causes a strong major reflection but lacks the strong reverberation caused by metal. It is hypoechoic and so appears as a dark band on ultrasound. It is important to note that although polyethylene appears hypoechoic, similar to fluid, its acoustic properties (e.g., impedance) are very different. Consequently, its surface will always be apparent, even in the presence of an effusion.

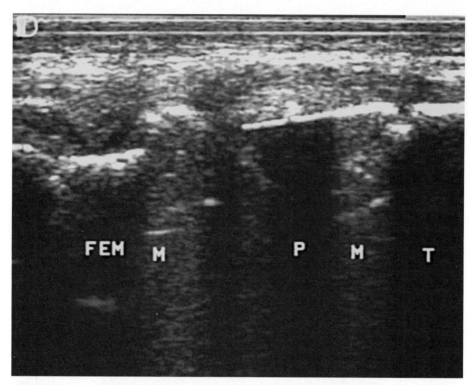

FIGURE 11–3   This is the ultrasound image of an intact arthroplasty. In order to appreciate the bone/metal/polyethylene interface, we recommend scanning on the longitudinal axis (the sagittal or coronal plane) across the joint. In this image, the ultrasound appearance of the cortical surface of the tibia (T), tibial tray (M), polyethylene spacer (P), femoral component (M), and femur (FEM) are seen from right to left. Again, the characteristic shadow/echo/shadow pattern indicating bone, metal, and polyethylene is apparent.

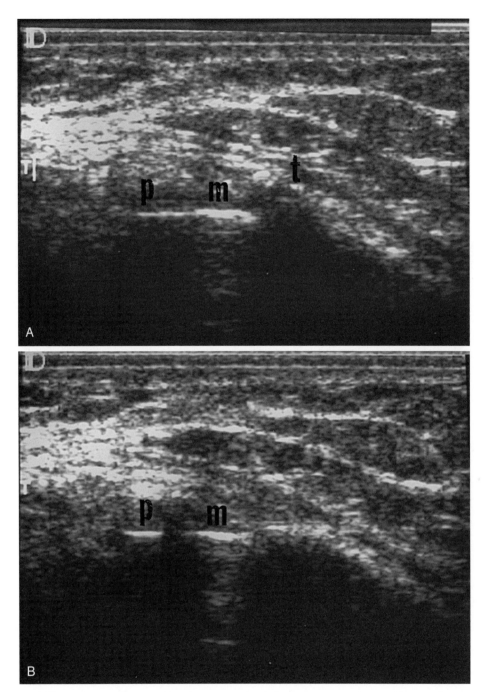

FIGURE 11-4 A horizontal split in a polyethylene spacer is shown. Two consecutive ultrasound images are presented moving from anterior to posterior in the medial compartment of a patient with a painful knee. **A:** The first image demonstrates an intact bone/metal/ polyethylene complex. Notice that the cortical margin of the tibia (t) is displaced slightly relative to the metallic echo (m). This is a normal finding, indicating that the tibial margin and the metallic tray are not flush on the plane on which the image is obtained. On this plane of imaging, the polyethylene spacer (p) is contiguous with the metallic tray (m). **B:** Subsequent images obtained more posteriorly demonstrate the development of a horizontal split in the polyethylene spacer along the axial plane. This is seen sonographically as an abrupt surface discontinuity in the third component of the shadow/echo/shadow complex, which corresponds to the polyethylene surface. The metallic tray (m) and the polyethylene spacer (p) are now separated by a hypoechoic gap.

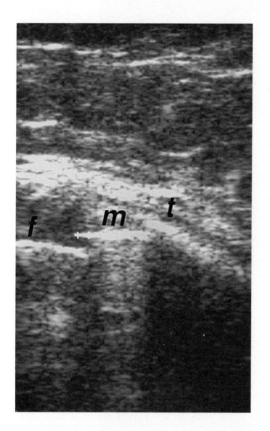

FIGURE 11–5 This image indicates complete loss of polyethylene. A sagittal ultrasound image obtained over the posterior aspect of the medial compartment shows a metal-on-metal appearance that is caused by the complete absence of polyethylene spacer. This appears as the absence of the hypoechoic band, corresponding to the third component of the shadow/echo/shadow complex. The metallic tibial tray (m) is on the right side of the image, adjacent to the tibial cortex (t), and the femoral component (f) is on the left. A small amount of residual polyethylene extends slightly beyond the femoral component.

FIGURE 11–6 This image indicates osteolysis at the bone/ metal interface and wear-debris synovitis in a patient with a painful knee. **A:** A coronal ultrasound image over the medial compartment of the left knee shows a large cyst-like erosion at the tibial bone/metal interface (arrow). There is focal loss of the tibial (T) echo along the cortical margin near the junction with the metallic tray (M). The arrow depicts the base of the erosion, which acts as a new reflective surface for the insonating ultrasound beam. **B:** A more anterior parasagittal ultrasound image of the medial compartment shows less pronounced erosion and widening of the bone/metal interface (T and M, respectively), and the gap and overlying anterior recess are filled with abnormal hypoechoic soft tissue. The erosion of the bone/metal interface is denoted by plus signs (+). The metallic tray is slightly displaced relative to the polyethylene spacer. In this plane of imaging, the polyethylene spacer is intact.

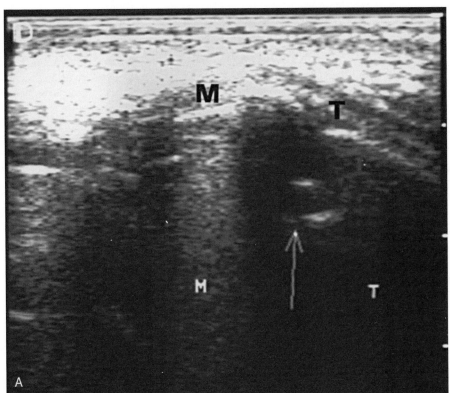

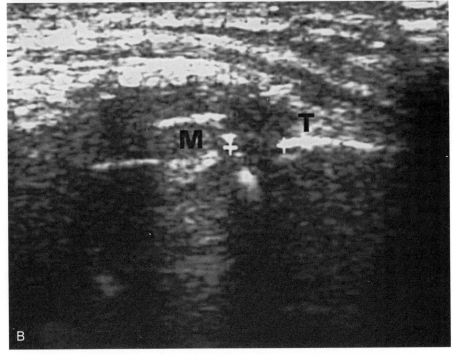

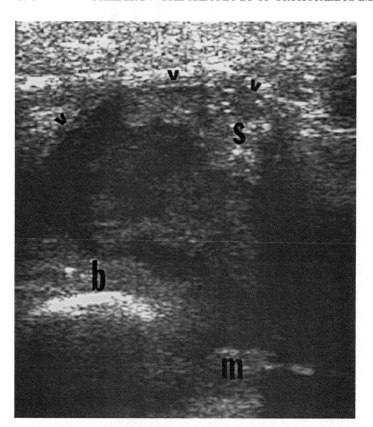

FIGURE 11–7 Wear-debris synovitis in a patient with arthroplasty and a painful knee is shown. A transverse ultrasound image obtained over the medial recess of the suprapatellar pouch reveals fluid, which appears completely black (anechoic), and nodular soft tissue (S) distending the pouch (v). The latter corresponds to nodular proliferative synovium and debris. The bone/metal interface (b and m, respectively) of the femur is located at the bottom of the image. Ultrasound provides a simple method of detecting fluid within the joint and periprosthetic collections of fluid (see Figs. 11–11 and 11–12) as well as a way of separating fluid from solid components. Likewise, the real-time nature of ultrasound provides a simple method of guiding the localization of needles for fluid aspiration and synovial biopsy (see Figs. 11–13 and 11–14).

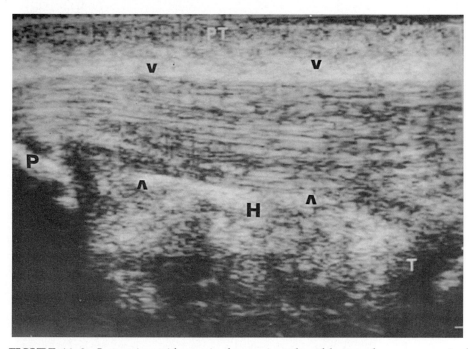

FIGURE 11–8 In a patient with anterior knee pain and total knee replacement, a sagittal midline ultrasound image obtained over the patella tendon (v) shows it to be enlarged and inhomogeneous, signs that are compatible with patellar tendinitis. Hoffa's fat pad (H) is the echogenic soft tissue below the tendon. The polyethylene spacer was shown to be intact on ultrasound examination. The presence of tendinosis, tendinitis, or tendon tears involving the extensor mechanism is easily evaluated on sonography. The patella (P) is the cortical echo at the left of the image. The anterior tibial tubercle (T) is not included on the image.

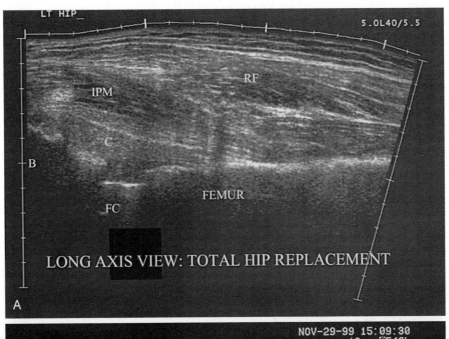

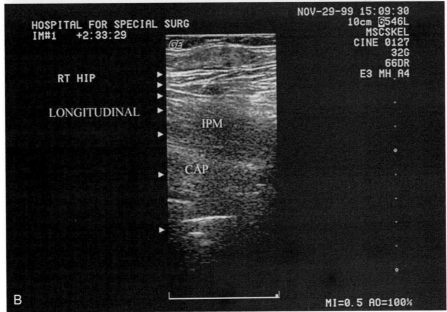

FIGURE 11–9 This figure reveals the ultrasound appearance of an intact total hip replacement. **A:** A longitudinal, extended-field-of-view ultrasound image was obtained along the proximal anterior thigh at the level of the joint prosthesis. The rectus femoris (RF) and iliopsoas (IPM) muscles are evident. Muscles normally appear hypoechoic, as these do, with interspersed echogenic linear echoes corresponding to the fibroadipose septa between muscle fascicles. The cortical surfaces of the native femur and supra-acetabular bone (B) present as well-marginated specular reflectors at the bottom of the image. In particular, the proximal femoral diaphysis should appear as a relatively smoothly marginated, continuous reflector. Portions of the intra-articular metallic femoral stem (FC) and acetabular component are evident. The pseudocapsule (C) appears as a thick echogenic band of tissue overlying the joint just deep to the iliopsoas muscle (IPM). Extended-field-of-view imaging is an example of newer ultrasound technology that effectively allows imaging over a large anatomic region. This is a useful feature for depicting anatomic relationships and the extent of an abnormality. **B:** A longitudinal ultrasound image was obtained over an intact hip arthroplasty using a small field of view. Again, the iliopsoas muscle (IPM) and pseudocapsule (CAP) can be seen. The bright linear echoes below the pseudocapsule correspond to the visualized femoral and acetabular components. Small-field-of-view imaging is the conventional manner in which ultrasound images are obtained. Images are acquired in real time and are of high resolution. Imaging may be performed during provocative maneuvers such as hip flexion and may provide real-time guidance for needle placement during ultrasound-guided interventions.

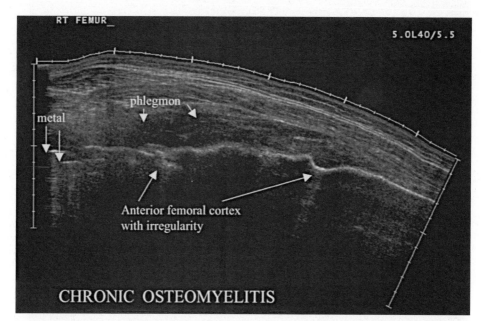

FIGURE 11–10 In a patient with a hip replacement and chronic osteomyelitis, a longitudinal, extended-field-of-view ultrasound image was obtained along the proximal anterior thigh at the level of the joint prosthesis and femoral diaphysis. The intra-articular metallic components (metal) are at the far left of the image. The anterior cortex of the femoral diaphysis demonstrates areas of irregularity (arrows) that presumably are related to small erosions with possible sinus tract formation. Immediately overlying this abnormal bone, there is a hypo-echoic area (arrows) that corresponds with an inflammatory mass (phlegmon) arising from the underlying osteomyelitis. The mass slightly displaces the overlying rectus femoris muscle anteriorly.

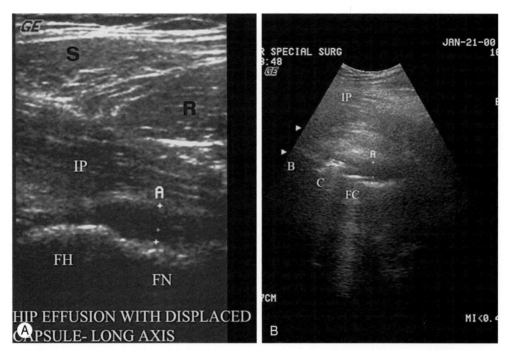

FIGURE 11–11 These images indicate the presence of hip effusions. **A:** A longitudinal ultrasound image was obtained over the native hip in a patient with rheumatoid arthritis. Portions of the sartorius (S), rectus femoris (R), and iliopsoas (IP) muscles are evident. Immediately below the iliopsoas muscle is a thick echogenic stripe corresponding to the joint capsule. The echogenic cortical reflector at the bottom of the image that shows posterior shadowing depicts the femoral head (FH) and femoral neck (FN), respectively. Normally, the capsule parallels the femoral neck with, at most, a thin hypoechoic line separating the bone from the overlying capsule. In this case, hypoechoic fluid displaces the anterior capsule, which forms a convex surface relative to the underlying femur. The distance A denotes the ultrasound measurement typically used to assess joint effusions. Normally, this value does not exceed 4 mm. In this case, the degree of capsular distension was more than 1 cm, indicating a moderately sized effusion. **B:** Similar principles apply in a patient with a total hip replacement. In this case, it is the pseudocapsule rather than the native capsule that is displaced. In this sagittal ultrasound image obtained over the anterior hip, the degree of distension (A) measures approximately 1.5 cm, indicating a moderately sized joint effusion. The fluid is situated between the pseudocapsule and portions of the intra-articular metallic components (C, FC) as well as a small segment of the native femur. B and IP refer to native acetabulum and iliopsoas muscle, respectively.

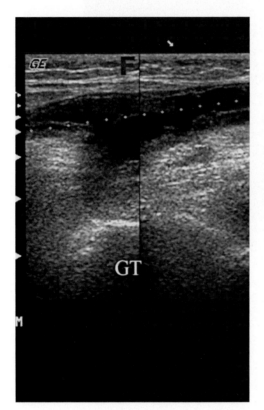

FIGURE 11–12   Extra-articular fluid collection in a patient with total hip replacement is pictured. The initial ultrasound image obtained over the anterior recess of the hip showed no significant joint effusion. This patient had a sensitive erythematous region over the greater trochanteric region of the hip. An ultrasound image obtained on the coronal plane at this location demonstrates a large collection immediately deep to the subcutaneous fat (F). This collection extends deeper into the soft tissues and is in direct contiguity with the greater trochanter (GT). No communication with the adjacent joint could be demonstrated. Fluid was aspirated under ultrasound guidance to achieve decompression as well as pathologic evaluation. The ability of ultrasound to directly localize for aspiration is illustrated in Figures 11–13 and 11–14.

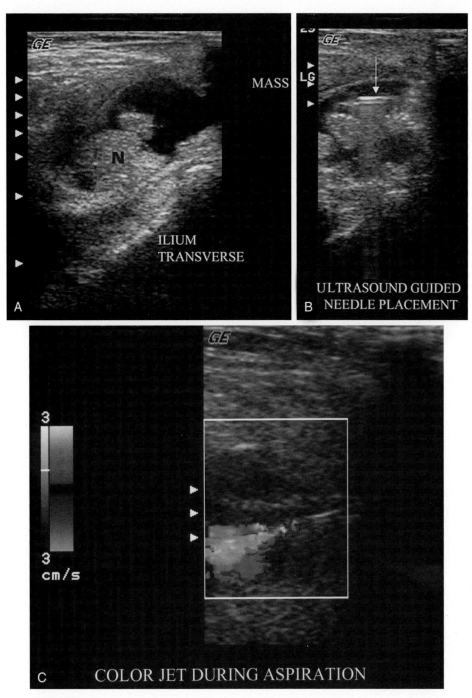

FIGURE 11–13 On physical examination of a patient with advanced osteoarthrosis being evaluated for left total hip replacement, a palpable mass was detected over the left groin, and it extended into the iliac fossa. Computed tomography demonstrated a large multiloculated cystic mass in relation to the iliopsoas muscle and in direct contiguity with the left hip. A large iliopsoas bursa was suggested. The patient was referred for ultrasound-guided aspiration of the mass. **A:** An ultrasound image obtained over the left iliac fossa in the axial plane demonstrates a complex mass containing nodular soft tissue (N) and anechoic (black) fluid. The mass overlies the iliacus muscle and iliac bone (ILIUM TRANSVERSE). **B:** An ultrasound image on the same plane shows the appearance of the metallic needle (arrow) with its characteristic reverberation artifact situated within the fluid component of the mass, anterior to the solid component. In this manner it was possible to ensure that the fluid component of the mass was being aspirated, rather than obtaining a negative aspirate because the needle was instead embedded in solid tissue. **C:** A transverse color Doppler sonogram obtained during aspiration of the mass causes a color jet to be directed toward the needle tip. The particulate nature of the fluid component is often evident on real-time examination as the presence of small echoes traveling toward the needle. These produce a Doppler shift detectable on color-flow imaging, as in this case.

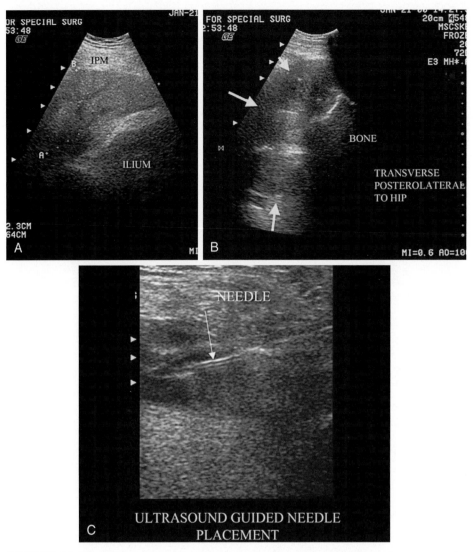

FIGURE 11–14 These are images of a patient with a right total hip replacement and a palpable mass over the right lower quadrant and gluteal region. The patient was sent for ultrasound evaluation and possible aspiration. **A:** An ultrasound image obtained on the parasagittal plane at the level of the right ilium shows the expansion of the underlying muscle (IPM), which is enlarged and echogenic. There is loss of normal distinction between the hypoechoic fascicles and the interspersed fibroadipose septa (see Fig. 11–11A). A fluid component is not evident in this image. **B:** An ultrasound image obtained on the axial plane, lateral to the ilium (BONE), demonstrates a similar echogenic appearance of the gluteal muscles (arrow). **C:** In this ultrasound image, a needle (arrow) is positioned into a more hypoechoic component of the mass. Again, the strong reverberations below the shaft of the needle may be noted. Old blood was aspirated, suggesting that this mass corresponds with infiltrative hematoma. The high density of the mass was demonstrated on subsequent noncontrast computed tomography, which is consistent with diffuse hemorrhage. Laboratory studies confirmed a recent drop in hematocrit.

Summary

These examples have shown that ultrasound provides an excellent method for evaluating the periprosthetic soft tissues of patients who have total joint replacements. Arthroplasty components present a characteristic appearance on ultrasound that can provide useful information regarding the integrity or loosening of components. Furthermore, ultrasound provides a technique for directly detecting periprosthetic fluid collections and joint effusions without the presence of metal-related artifacts. The real-time nature of ultrasound enables both the performance of provocative maneuvers during imaging and the provision of guidance for aspiration or biopsy. With these capabilities, ultrasound can play an important role in assessing a patient with a painful total joint replacement.

REFERENCES

1. Yashar AA, Adler RS, Grady-Benson JC, et al. An ultrasound method to evaluate polyethylene component wear in total knee replacement arthroplasty. Am J Ortho 1996;25:702–704.
2. Van Holsbeeck MT, Eyler WR, Sherman LS, et al. Detection of infection in loosened hip prostheses: efficacy of sonography. Am J Roentgen 1994;163:381–384.

12

—

Nuclear Medicine Imaging

——

ADAM W. J. TONAKIE

RICHARD WAHL

Scintigraphic evaluation of orthopedic implants is usually performed to investigate suspected postoperative complications, including the detection of radiologically occult fractures (such as stress fractures resulting from increased mobilization), the staging of the maturation of heterotopic bone formation, and the assessment of possible loosening or infection. Nuclear medicine studies are generally much more sensitive than plain radiographs, and their interpretation is typically not significantly compromised by the presence of orthopedic hardware as are computed tomography and magnetic resonance imaging.

Triple-phase bone scans using a technetium-labeled diphosphonate are universally used in the assessment of heterotopic bone and suspected stress fractures, but a number of other imaging techniques, using a variety of radiopharmaceuticals, have also been employed in the investigation and differentiation of loosening and infection. These techniques include the bone scan and its variations, the gallium scan, the indium- or technetium-labeled white blood cell (WBC) scan, combinations of the above and, most recently, dual-labeled WBC sulfur colloid marrow scans. These various approaches have arisen in attempts to overcome a perennial problem: nuclear medicine skeletal imaging studies offer excellent sensitivity but poor specificity.

Both blood-flow and osteoblastic activity dictate uptake of diphosphonates. A triple-phase bone scan increases the specificity of the study, as hyperemia is typically associated with acute, rather than mature, heterotopic bone formation; acute stress fractures and infection but not loosening; and postoperative and degenerative changes, all of which may show increased activity on delayed imaging.

Phase one, the radionuclide angiogram, or blood-flow phase, is acquired as dynamic 2- to 5-second images for 60 seconds after bolus intravenous injection, preferably in an arm vein, when investigating arthroplasties in lower limbs. It evaluates the vascular delivery of the tracer to the region of interest. The second phase, the blood-pool or soft-tissue phase, depicts a combination of flow, regional tissue extraction, and distribution volume effects. Images are obtained immediately after the flow study, typically over a 5-minute period or for a certain number of counts, usually 200 to 300 K for the appendicular skeleton. Both sides are always imaged so a comparison can be made between the symptomatic and asymptomatic joints. Delayed third-phase static images, which reflect tracer retained by avid chemisorption sites in the bone, are acquired 2 to 4 hours after injection (following bladder emptying, particularly if the hips are being evaluated). Single photon emission computed tomography (SPECT) imaging is performed at this time, if indicated. Further delayed imaging—a fourth phase—usually at 24 hours, is often performed to evaluate suspected osteomyelitis in the distal appendicular skeleton. This is most commonly indicated in a diabetic patient with poor peripheral blood flow and commonly compromised renal function, both causes of delayed uptake by bone, but is rarely required for the assessment of more proximal arthroplasties.

Acute fractures that occur during arthroplasty surgery or as stress injuries resulting from increased mobility after arthroplasty are typically identified as focal areas of increased activity on the blood-pool and delayed phases of the bone scan. Heterotopic ossification can be diagnosed scintigraphically prior to its appearance on plain radiographs. The three-phase bone scan can also be used to determine optimal timing for surgical intervention, as the condition may recur if surgery is performed prior to the maturation of the ossification. The process is immature when increased activity is present in all phases; increased uptake only on delayed images signifies maturation (Figs. 12–1 and 12–2).

The investigation and differentiation of loosening and infection by means of bone scans is more problematic for several reasons. First, there is considerable variation in the intensity, distribution, and time course of technetium-labeled diphosphonate uptake in asymptomatic patients postoperatively. Second, both the type of prosthesis used and the joint involved influence the pattern and temporal course of normal postoperative uptake. In asymptomatic patients, 90% of those with cemented total hip prostheses have a normal scan 1 year postoperatively, whereas after total

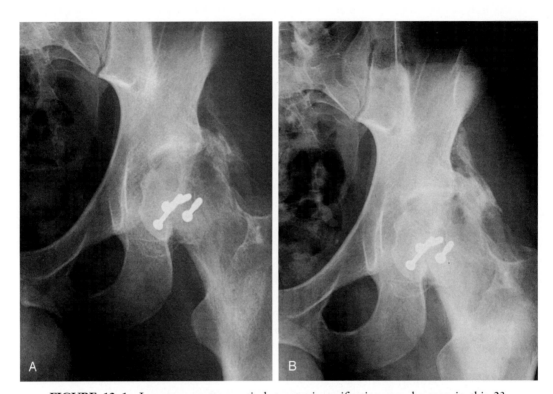

FIGURE 12–1 Immature posttraumatic heterotopic ossification may be seen in this 23-year-old male patient who was involved in a motor vehicle accident in which he suffered a left femoral head dislocation and fracture; it was internally fixed with lag screws. **A:** A plain radiograph of the left hip obtained 2 months later demonstrates the development of heterotopic ossification. **B:** The ossification has shown significant progression in the follow-up study performed 4 months later.

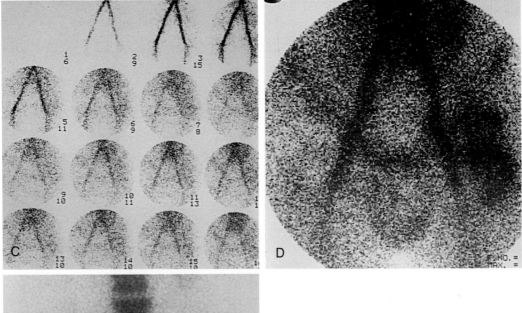

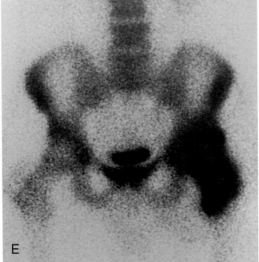

FIGURE 12–1 *Continued.* **C, D,** and **E:** A triple-phase bone scan was performed 6 months later to stage the maturity of the ossification process, with a view to planning surgical resection. Increased activity is clearly evident over the left hip in the first two phases of the study, the radionuclide angiogram (C) and the blood pool (D). This is indicative of the immaturity of the process. Surgery should therefore be delayed to reduce the risk of recurrence. Delayed images (E) show intense uptake in the heterotopic bone, which was severely restricting movement of the hip.

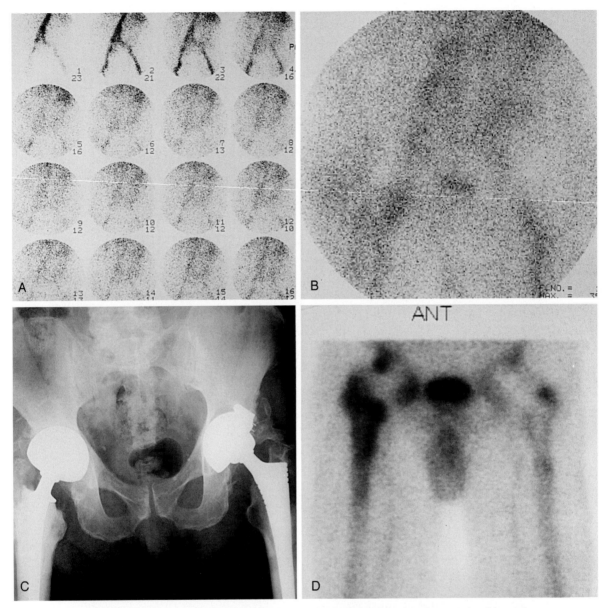

FIGURE 12–2 Mature posttraumatic heterotopic ossification may be seen in this triple-phase bone scan of a 72-year-old male patient who had had bilateral total hip arthroplasties. An uncemented prosthesis had been inserted on the left 9 years before this study and was asymptomatic. The right arthroplasty had been originally performed 3 months prior to this study but had been revised after 2 weeks because of instability. Two years later the patient presented with persistent right hip pain. Investigation revealed an elevated erythrocyte sedimentation rate, and although an arthrogram demonstrated no evidence of loosening, an aspiration culture performed at the time tested positive for *Staphylococcus aureus*. **A:** The blood flow study shows subtly increased activity in the right hip. **B:** The activity is more obvious in the second phase. **C:** There is no increased activity in these phases in the mature heterotopic ossification of the left hip, as is demonstrated in the pelvic radiograph. **D:** The delayed image shows intense, diffusely increased tracer accumulation around both the femoral and the acetabular components on the infected right side; it shows less intense focal uptake in the region of both the greater trochanter and the tip of the femoral prosthesis on the asymptomatic left side. The femoral prosthesis is defined by the photopenic central region.

knee arthroplasty, approximately 90% of those with tibial components (Fig. 12–3) and 60% of those with femoral components show increased periprosthetic activity more than 1 year postoperatively. In fact, the natural course of a total knee arthroplasty is to demonstrate mildly to moderately increased activity for years, and truly quiescent scans are unusual. Persisting activity in the hip occurs most commonly around the greater trochanter and the distal tip of the prosthesis (see Fig. 12–2C). As cementless, porous-coated implants are designed to stimulate osteoblastic activity and hence new bone growth around and into the pores of the prosthesis, uptake patterns are more variable in distribution and more prevalent after 1 year than they are in patients with the cemented variety. In contrast, a smooth-surfaced, cementless prosthesis lacks pores and is not designed to elicit an osteoblastic response. Instead, it has ridges and grooves that help to anchor it. The addition of a bone graft results in increased blastic activity and, hence, prolonged uptake on bone scans.

In the radionuclide evaluation of these complications of joint replacement, bone scintigraphy is probably most useful when the images are normal. A negative bone scan helps to rule out infections, but they are uncommon, and although a scan that shows persisting, intensely increased activity suggests loosening or infection, false-positive rates are high, as this increased periprosthetic activity may reflect only variable postoperative changes. This highlights the major limitation of bone scans. Even utilizing the three-phase technique, there is good sensitivity for detecting complications, but poor specificity.

Furthermore, not only is there poor specificity in distinguishing between normal and pathologic postoperative uptake, there is also difficulty in separating loosening alone from loosening secondary to infection. Loosening may be asymptomatic and therefore not clinically important; however, if there are symptoms and signs of loosening, infection must always be excluded. Infection occurs in up to 4% of total hip arthroplasties, in less than 0.5% of primary total knee arthroplasties, and in significantly more revisions. Obviously, its presence alters management. Evidence of increased activity in the blood-flow and pool phases in the majority of cases of infection was thought to be useful in its differentiation from loosening, in which only the delayed images supposedly demonstrate increased uptake. However, recent studies suggest that in contrast to osteomyelitis in general, three-phase bone scans do little to improve the accuracy of routine bone scanning for diagnosing infected joint replacements. Continued attempts to improve the specificity of bone scintigraphy, particularly in the hip, have addressed the pattern of periprosthetic uptake. Focal periprosthetic uptake was reported to be typical of loosening, whereas a diffuse pattern was most likely to be associated with infection. Further reports, however, have not supported this assertion, and some have, in fact, contradicted it. Although the uptake is usually more intense in cases of infection, focal or diffuse patterns of increased uptake around the prosthesis on delayed images can be seen soon after operation with both loosening and infection as well as with normal healing.

Because of the inherent problem of poor specificity, other radionuclide techniques have been used instead of or in addition to the bone scan. One approach to increasing specificity for the detection of loosening has been to perform simultaneous bone scans and nuclear arthrograms. After 2- to 3-hour delayed bone scan images have been obtained, either indium In 111 or technetium Tc 99m sulfur colloid is injected along with iodinated contrast for a dual arthrogram. Flow of the injected radiopharmaceutical around the stem of a femoral component is indicative of loosening in the hip.

Gallium was developed as a bone-seeking radiopharmaceutical but was first used clinically to image tumors. Its ability to localize at sites of infection and inflammation was soon noted and utilized. Gallium binds to transferrin and is thus transported to sites of inflammation or infection. Although the precise mechanism of localization is not known, an adequate blood supply increases vascular permeability, bacterial uptake, and binding to leukocytes and released lactoferrin; all are thought to play a role.

Drawbacks of gallium imaging include its four photopeaks, the required delay

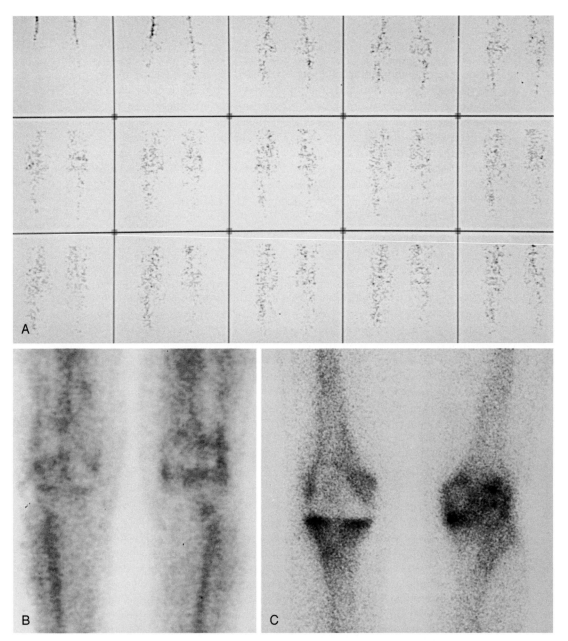

FIGURE 12–3 Combined scans are taken to exclude periprosthetic infection. A 73-year-old male patient presented with knee pain that had been present since a revision, 1 year earlier, of a right total knee arthroplasty with an uncemented prosthesis. The original arthroplasty had been performed 12 years prior to this study. A triple-phase bone scan was performed. **A:** The flow is normal. **B:** The blood-pool study shows only subtle activity in the proximal tibia just below the tibial prosthesis, and it is less intense than that in the contralateral knee. **C** through **F:** Anterior, posterior, medial, and lateral delayed scans demonstrate diffusely increased activity in the proximal tibia adjacent to the prosthesis; this is seen as a photopenic defect, along with abnormal uptake in the left knee, particularly in its medial compartment. The pattern of activity on the left is typical of degenerative joint disease. The normal first two phases of the study in the symptomatic right knee are suggestive of normal postoperative uptake, but loosening, with or without infection, could not be definitely excluded, and further studies were therefore performed. **G:** A scan of the white blood cells using indium In 111 labeling demonstrated subtly increased tracer accumulation in the right distal femur and proximal tibia when compared to the left. **H:** Therefore, a technetium Tc 99m sulfur colloid marrow scan was performed to determine the normal distribution of marrow. Comparison of the two studies shows almost exactly concordant uptake, indicating that the asymmetry in activity is due to the presence of normal marrow, not infection.

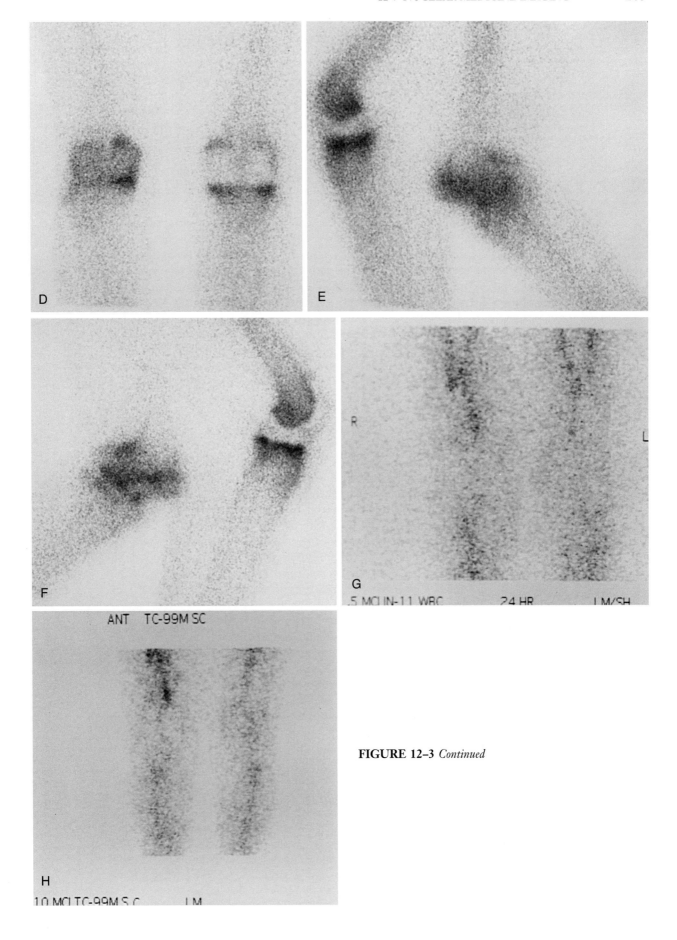

FIGURE 12–3 *Continued*

until scanning D, usually 24 and 48 hours, and its renal and intestinal excretion. With respect to orthopedic imaging, gallium scans suffer from the same lack of specificity as do bone scans. Because of uptake by normal bone and possible increased activity in patients with prostheses, other previous surgery, fractures, or underlying bone disease, false-positive studies for osteomyelitis occur. Sequential gallium studies of bone were therefore introduced and were found to be most useful when the scans were spatially incongruent or when the gallium study was negative. However, as these patterns are not common, the technique has been shown to result in only a slight improvement over bone scintigraphy in isolation.

Scintigraphic imaging of infection using radiolabeled WBCs is physiologically appealing and is theoretically the best technique for diagnosing infected joint replacements. This is because in the absence of infection, WBCs do not accumulate at sites of increased bone mineral turnover. Therefore, the poor specificity seen with bone scans, which results from uptake in noninfectious conditions, such as heterotopic ossification, metastatic disease, degenerative joint changes, and noninfective loosening, should not be encountered. Leukocytes can be labeled with either indium In 111 or technetium Tc 99m. Technical and imaging drawbacks include the long preparation time and exposure to blood products and, with indium, a comparatively long delay until imaging as well as poor count rates resulting from the small dose necessitated by high splenic dosimetry. Furthermore, though results have varied widely depending on the criteria used for a positive study, overall they have been generally disappointing. The chronic, low-grade inflammation present in these patients has been cited as one of several reasons for the reported low sensitivity and specificity.

Early reports on the diagnosis of infected orthopedic prostheses by means of the combination of labeled WBC and bone scans were promising, but further studies have been less enthusiastic. Problems encountered have in part arisen because diphosphonates are taken up by, and reflect conditions affecting, the bone. In contrast, labeled leukocyte accumulation is dictated by the status of the marrow. Processes that affect the marrow may not have a significant impact on the bone and vice versa.

The recent introduction of the dual-labeled WBC/sulfur colloid marrow scan has solved many of the problems encountered in interpreting the labeled WBC studies both in isolation and in combination with bone scans. The rationale for this technique is that the marrow scan increases the sensitivity of the WBC study by enabling discrimination between uptake in normal marrow, which may be ectopic in location, and foci of infection. Both studies depict radiotracer accumulation in the reticuloendothelial cells of the marrow. Infection results in decreased uptake of sulfur colloid and simultaneous stimulation of uptake of labeled leukocytes, which results in a discordant or incongruent pattern when the two studies are compared. Other factors that may influence marrow distribution include previous fracture or radiotherapy, Paget's disease, metastasis, hematologic diseases (such as sickle cell anemia and thalassemia), and joint replacement surgery. These processes have been shown to produce concordant patterns of either increased or decreased uptake.

The marrow scan is a comparatively simple procedure requiring no preparation of the patient. Images of the region of interest can be obtained beginning 10 minutes after the intravenous administration of 10 mCi of technetium Tc 99m sulfur colloid. Scans have consistently been above 90%, and this technique is currently the best radionuclide procedure for the diagnosis of an infected joint replacement.

Currently, the recommended approach to radionuclide diagnosis of an infected joint replacement and orthopedic hardware in general is as follows. Labeled leukocyte imaging should be performed first because if no periprosthetic activity is present, the study is negative for infection and scintigraphic investigation is complete. If activity is present, then marrow imaging should be performed, and if images are congruent, the study is negative; incongruent images and activity on the labeled WBC study but not on the marrow study are positive for infection (Figs. 12–4 through 12–7).

Text continued on page 211

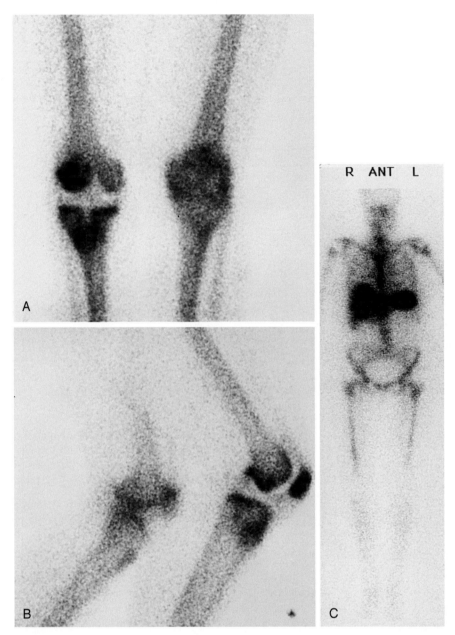

FIGURE 12–4 An uninfected but painful arthroplasty is shown. This 72-year-old female developed pain following a right total knee arthroplasty 4 years earlier. Plain radiographs were normal, so a triple-phase bone scan was performed. Blood-flow and -pool images (not shown) indicated subtly increased activity in the right knee around the patella and proximal tibia. **A** and **B:** Delayed scanning showed concordantly increased activity in these areas, which is a nonspecific finding. **C:** To increase specificity, a WBC study with indium In 111 labeling was requested. There is subtle asymmetry in marrow activity in both the distal femur and the proximal tibia, but there is no correlate for the increased patellar activity demonstrated on the bone scan. Thus, there are no findings to suggest infection. Indium-labeled leukocytes normally accumulate in the liver and spleen and in hematopoietically active marrow. In the normal adult population, such marrow is typically confined to the axial skeleton and the proximal humeri and femurs. However, many conditions, including prosthetic surgery, can result in alterations in this normal pattern. In such circumstances, separating ectopic normal functioning marrow from infection is problematic, and false positives are unavoidable unless a technetium Tc 99m sulfur colloid marrow imaging study is also performed.

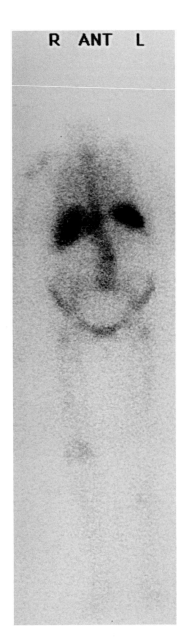

FIGURE 12–5 An infected arthroplasty was discovered in this patient. After 3 to 4 days of weakness and deteriorating overall status, this 81-year-old female with a history of severe rheumatoid arthritis and bilateral total knee arthroplasties was admitted following a lumbar puncture that revealed a diagnosis of bacterial meningitis. She developed pain and swelling in the right knee, so a white blood cell study with indium In 111 labeling was performed. It demonstrated multifocal increased uptake involving the right knee, the right shoulder, and the left mid tibia. An arthrotomy was performed on the right knee and pus was drained from it. An ultrasound-guided arthrocentesis of the shoulder obtained noninflammatory fluid.

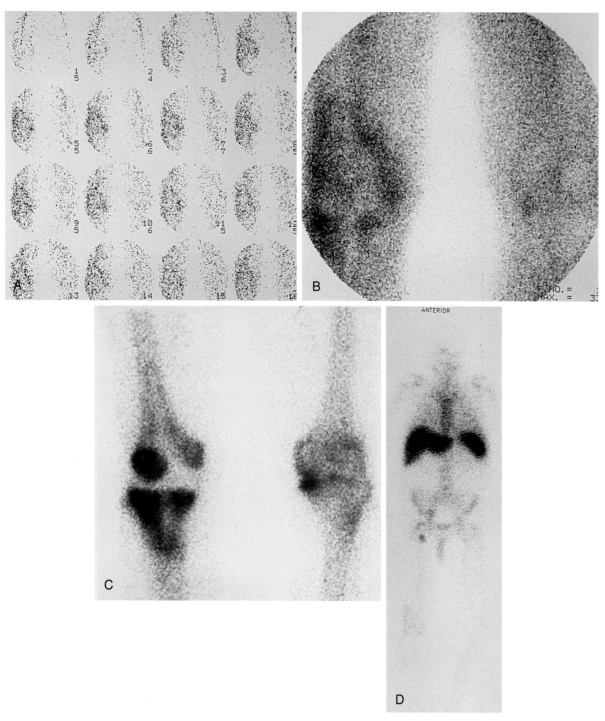

FIGURE 12–6 An infected arthroplasty that includes reactive lymph nodes is shown. A 71-year-old patient presented with progressively increasing pain and decreasing range of motion in the right knee after a fall. He had a right total knee arthroplasty 4 years previously, and it had been revised 2 years later. Examination revealed a swollen, tender joint, and blood work showed an elevated erythrocyte sedimentation rate. Plain radiographs showed good alignment and no evidence of loosening or infection, but some patellar subluxation had occurred. Scintigraphic investigations included a bone scan and a white blood cell study with indium In 111 labeling. The bone scan was strongly positive in all phases: **A:** Flow; **B:** Blood pool; **C:** Delayed. These findings are consistent with a diagnosis of infection. **D:** To increase specificity, a labeled leukocyte study was performed.

Illustration continued on following page

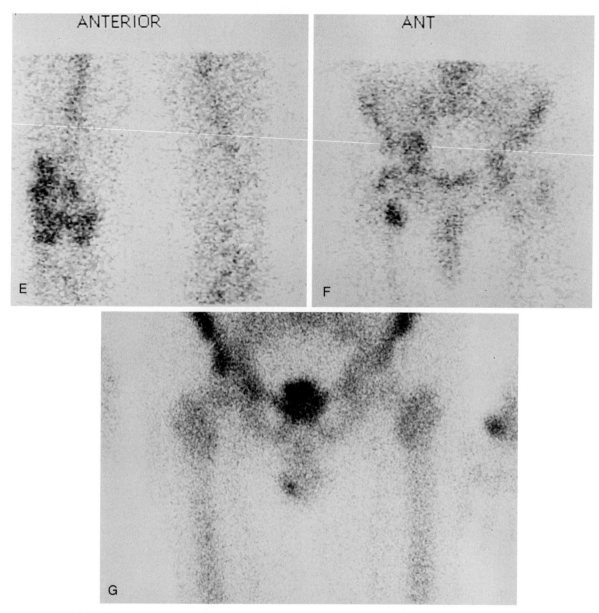

FIGURE 12–6 *Continued.* **E:** It demonstrated congruent increased uptake in the knee. **F:** Further foci were revealed in the right groin and pelvis. **G:** The inguinal and pelvic foci were not identified on the bone scan. The soft-tissue uptake almost certainly represented activity in reactive lymph nodes. On the spot images of the pelvis and knees, the increased uptake in the superior and medial acetabulum is typical of degenerative change, as is the activity in the medial compartment of the left knee. Joint aspiration was positive for *Staphylococcus* species, and purulent material was present at operation.

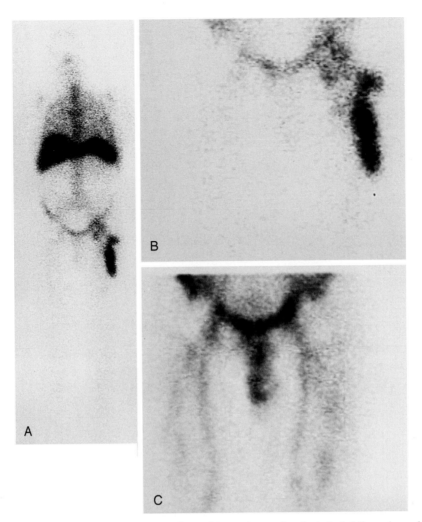

FIGURE 12–7 Infection was found in this patient who had had bilateral total hip arthroplasties several years before these scans. The left side had become infected and was revised. Pain recurred and increased; the patient became mildly febrile, and radiographs demonstrated loosening of the femoral prosthesis. **A:** A labeled leukocyte study was performed to ascertain whether the loosening was associated with recurrent infection. **B:** There is intense tracer accumulation around the left femoral prosthesis. **C:** The patient had had previous surgery so a technetium Tc 99m sulfur colloid marrow scan was performed to evaluate for any significant alteration of the expected normal marrow distribution. Comparison of the two studies reveals obvious discordance, which indicates that the cause of the abnormal white cell accumulation is infection rather than an alteration in the marrow distribution subsequent to surgery. A labeled scan of the white blood cells should be the first scintigraphic investigation performed if infection of a replaced joint is suspected. If the results are normal, infection can be excluded as the cause, but if there is increased uptake, a sulfur colloid marrow scan should be performed. Congruent studies rule out infection in the vast majority of cases; discordant scans increase the specificity of a white cell study alone and facilitate a confident diagnosis of infection.

BIBLIOGRAPHY

Palestro CJ. Chronic infection: radionuclide diagnosis of the infected joint replacement. In Murray IPC, Ell PJ, eds. Nuclear Medicine in Clinical Diagnosis and Treatment, Vol. 2. Edinburgh: Churchill-Livingstone, 1994.

Palestro CJ. Radionuclide imaging after skeletal interventional procedures. Semin Nucl Med 1995;25:3–14.

13

—

Foot and Ankle
Implants

SHIRLEY CHOW
CHARLES L. SALTZMAN
GEORGES Y. EL-KHOURY

Arthroplasty and arthrodesis are performed in the foot and ankle for various indications, including painful osteoarthritis secondary to trauma or inflammatory arthritis and posttraumatic, acquired, or developmental deformities.

Total ankle replacements are now performed for limited indications, specifically in patients with rheumatoid arthritis or posttraumatic arthritis and limited activity needs.[1, 2] There are two general types of ankle prostheses: semiconstrained (Fig. 13–1), which allows only dorsal and plantar flexion, and nonconstrained (Fig. 13–2). Preoperatively, there should be ankle stability[3] and adequate bone stock for prosthetic support.[1, 4] With weightbearing, the tibial and talar components should be parallel to each other and to the floor. On the lateral radiograph, the tibial component angles posteroinferiorly.[4] Complications of total ankle replacements include periprosthetic fracture; loosening or infection; subsidence of the implants; and impingement, most commonly between the lateral malleolus and talus.[2, 4, 5]

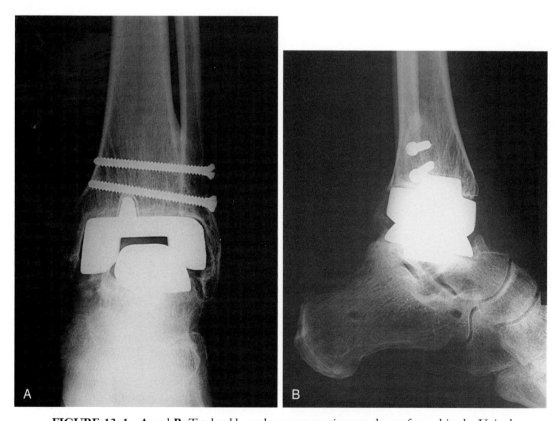

FIGURE 13–1 A and **B:** Total ankle replacement continues to be performed in the United States on a selective basis. Two current models are utilized: the Agility Ankle (DePuy, Wausau, IN) requires the fusion of the tibiofibular syndesmosis in order to obtain stability of the tibial component. Subsidence of the talar component is independent of the syndesmosis fusion. The circumferential lucent line around the tibial component suggests fibrous ingrowth and lack of bony union. Despite this, early clinical results with use of this implant are encouraging.

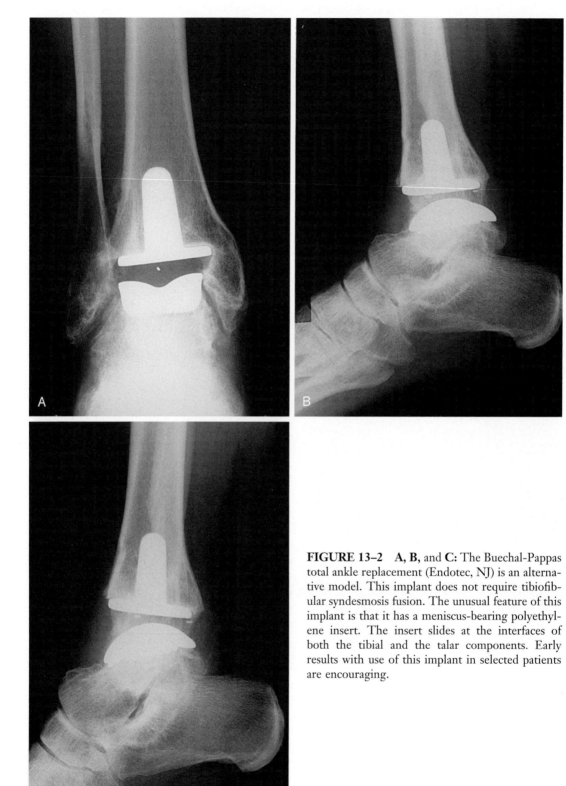

FIGURE 13–2   A, B, and **C:** The Buechal-Pappas total ankle replacement (Endotec, NJ) is an alternative model. This implant does not require tibiofibular syndesmosis fusion. The unusual feature of this implant is that it has a meniscus-bearing polyethylene insert. The insert slides at the interfaces of both the tibial and the talar components. Early results with use of this implant in selected patients are encouraging.

Ankle fusion can be performed primarily (Fig. 13–3), most commonly for posttraumatic or secondary osteoarthritis or to salvage failed arthroplasty. The tibial and talar articular surfaces are resected, bone graft is placed, and screws, plates, pins, staples, or clamps are placed for fixation. The foot should be fused in neutral position.[5-7] Again, the talar dome should be parallel to the floor. Persistent joint lucency with surrounding sclerosis that is present beyond 6 months after arthroplasty is a sign of nonunion (Fig. 13–4). With loss of ankle motion, secondary arthritis may develop in the midfoot and hindfoot.[7]

When the subtalar joint is also diseased, combined tibiotalocalcaneal arthrodesis can be performed (see Fig. 13–4). Fixation is made with large screws or an intramedullary nail.[8] Because the nail is inserted retrograde through the heel, injury to the nerve to the abductor digiti quinti, a branch of the lateral plantar nerve, may cause persistent heel pain.[9]

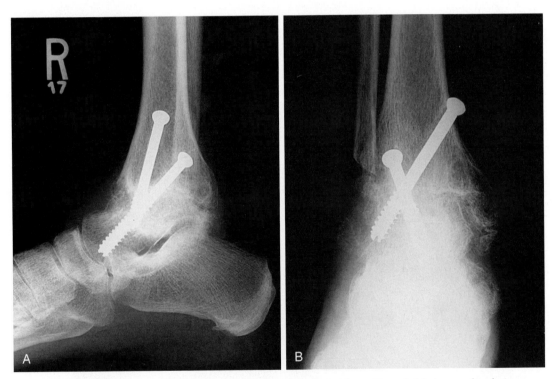

FIGURE 13–3   A and **B:** The primary surgical treatment for ankle arthritis is an arthrodesis procedure. The goal of the procedure is to obtain a stable tibiotalar fusion in good alignment. The optimal position is neutral in the sagittal plane, 5 degrees of valgus and 5 to 15 degrees of external rotation. Rigid internal fixation with screws or screws and plate assemblies improves the likelihood of fusion. Resection of the lateral malleolus improves cosmesis and removes the possibility of continued pain at the talofibular articulation.

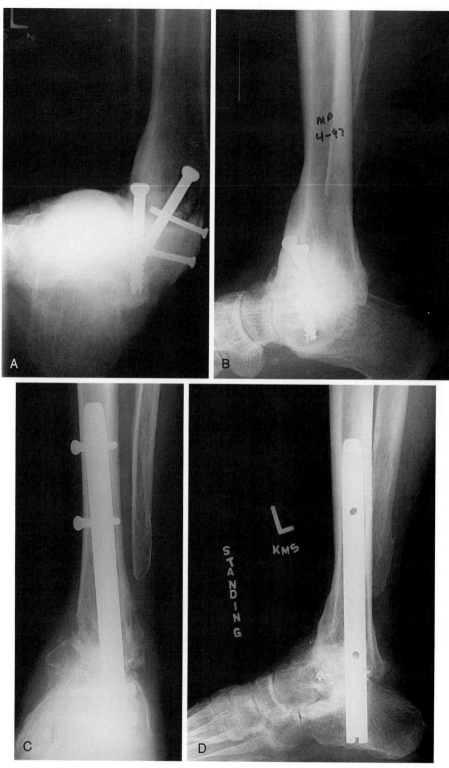

FIGURE 13–4 Occasionally, ankle fusions develop nonunions and then displace. Factors that contribute to this are unrecognized neuropathic arthropathy, tobacco usage, and screw fixation techniques that allow poor rotational control of the construct. **A** and **B:** In the case in this image, the nonunion of the ankle went on to become a severe valgus deformity. **C** and **D:** Arthrodesis of the tibiotalocalcaneal articulations was necessary to achieve stability. A large, locked, reamed, intramedullary nail was used to maintain the reduction.

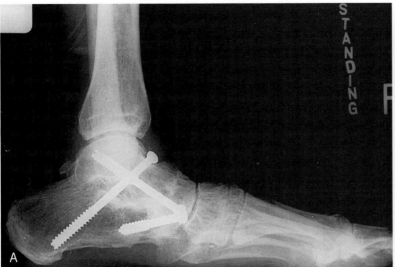
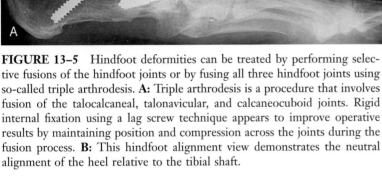
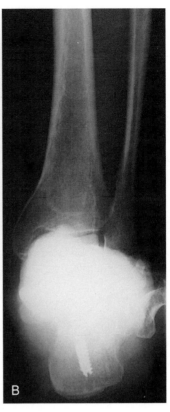

FIGURE 13–5 Hindfoot deformities can be treated by performing selective fusions of the hindfoot joints or by fusing all three hindfoot joints using so-called triple arthrodesis. **A:** Triple arthrodesis is a procedure that involves fusion of the talocalcaneal, talonavicular, and calcaneocuboid joints. Rigid internal fixation using a lag screw technique appears to improve operative results by maintaining position and compression across the joints during the fusion process. **B:** This hindfoot alignment view demonstrates the neutral alignment of the heel relative to the tibial shaft.

Common indications for subtalar and talonavicular arthrodesis are deformity after calcaneal fractures[7] and painful, acquired flatfoot,[10] respectively. Triple arthrodesis (Fig. 13–5) is indicated when there are combined midfoot and hindfoot deformities and when a salvage procedure is necessary.[11] Preoperatively, there must be stability of the ankle for these procedures. After triple arthrodesis, the hindfoot should be in a neutral or slight valgus position (see Fig. 13–5).[12] Complications of triple arthrodesis include nonunion (especially of the talonavicular joint), osteonecrosis of the talus,[7] secondary arthritis of the ankle or distal joints, and recurrent collapse.[11]

Acquired deformities of the forefoot can be painful and disfiguring and can alter weightbearing, resulting in callus formation, ulcers, and stress fractures.

Hallux valgus is one of the most common foot deformities. It is most often seen in women and is largely due to mismatch between the foot structure and "fashionable" shoe design. It may be associated with metatarsus varus or flatfoot deformities. Normally, angulation between the proximal phalanx and metatarsal should be 15 degrees valgus; similarly, the angle between the first and second metatarsal axes should be approximately 9 degrees. With increasing hallux valgus, bunion formation (prominent medial eminence of the first metatarsal) and uncovering of the sesamoids occur. Corrective procedures include resection of the medial eminence with soft-tissue realignment; various osteotomies of the proximal phalanx or head, neck, or base of the first metatarsal (Fig. 13–6); fusion of the tarsometatarsal joint (Fig. 13–7); and metatarsophalangeal (MTP) joint arthroplasty or arthrodesis (Fig. 13–8). Complications include nonunion; recurrence; excessive shortening of the first ray, which shifts load to the other metatarsals[7]; and arthritis of the first MTP joint.

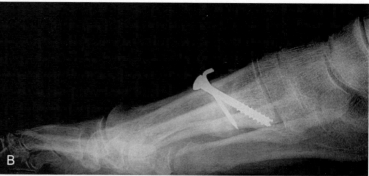

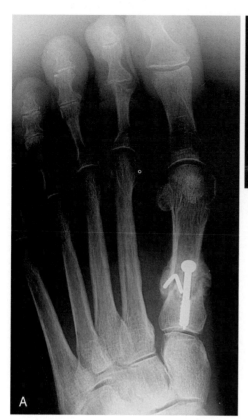

FIGURE 13–6 A variety of operations are utilized for the treatment of hallux valgus deformity. Perhaps the most common strategy involves performing an osteotomy of the first metatarsal. This case shows a hypertrophic delayed union of a proximal first metatarsal osteotomy. The reduction of the first MTP joint appears excellent on the anteroposterior radiograph, as restitution of the normal sesamoid–metatarsal relationship has occurred.

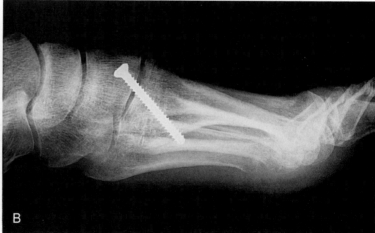

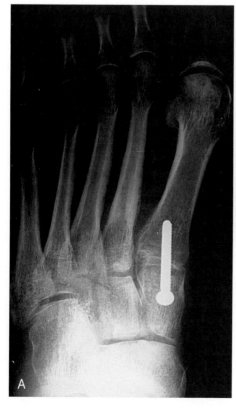

FIGURE 13–7 **A** and **B:** For patients with ligamentous laxity and hypermobility of the first metatarsal–cuneiform joint, arthrodesis of that joint is the preferred procedure. In this case, a single screw has fixed the first metatarsal–cuneiform arthrodesis site with resulting excellent realignment of the first MTP joint.

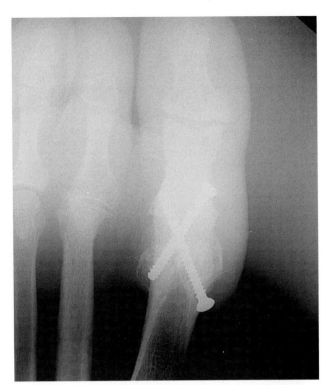

FIGURE 13–8 For patients with arthritis or severe deformity, a fusion of the first MTP joint may be the best treatment for hallux valgus. Crossed lag-screw fixation is one of the most stable mechanical constructs for holding this joint during the initial month of fusion. The patient in this image also demonstrates subluxation of the second MTP joint, which has not been reduced.

First MTP osteoarthritis (hallux rigidus) and flexion deformities of the toes at the proximal interphalangeal (IP) joint (hammer toe), distal IP joint (mallet toe), or both (cock-up toe) can be treated by arthroplasty (Fig. 13–9) or arthrodesis. Fixed dorsal subluxation of the metatarsals can be treated by partial resection of the metatarsal heads[7] or of the bases of the proximal phalanges.

Hallux valgus, hallux rigidis, and toe deformities, including arthritis, short toes, hammer toes, and failed arthrodeses may be treated by silicone implant arthroplasty.[7, 10] Implants are single- or double-stemmed, nonhinged or hinged. There should be adequate bone stock for implant support. For digital implants, there should be adequate vascular supply and longitudinal alignment of the toe and shaft size to fit the stem or stems; MTP joint deformities must be corrected.[13] The use of implants retains toe length (and thus distribution of load)[13, 14] and some mobility. Because of the frequently occurring complications, including silicone synovitis (Fig. 13–10), implant fracture or displacement (Fig. 13–11), and persistent swelling and loss of motion resulting from fibrosis around the implant and joint,[4, 7, 10] silicone implants are now rarely performed in foot surgery.

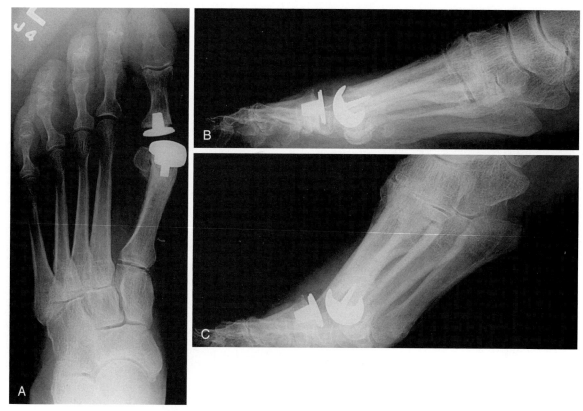

FIGURE 13–9 A, B, and **C:** Anteroposterior, standing lateral, and forced dorsiflexion lateral views, respectively, of a metal polyethylene first MTP joint replacement. These replacements have been advocated in the treatment of osteoarthritis of the first MTP joint. Their use has fallen into disfavor because of relatively high rates of loosening and subsidence of the component. The patient in this image complained of postoperative bunion pain, which was probably related to the mismatch between this relatively large metatarsal head component and her native first metatarsal.

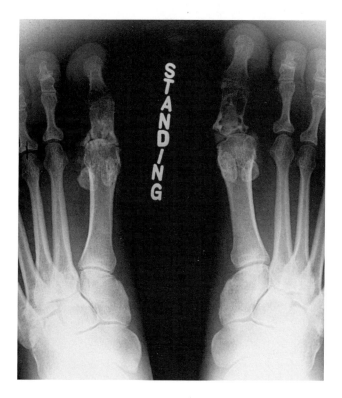

FIGURE 13–10 Silastic polymer implants have been widely used in the treatment of first MTP arthritis and, less commonly, for arthritic complaints in other areas of the forefoot. These implants have been plagued by fragmentation and breakdown and have caused regional osteolysis. The case in this image shows the results of using Silastic implants bilaterally at the first MTP joints. On the left, the implant has been removed after massive osteolysis and bony fragmentation. On the right, the implant remains intact although fragmented and causing local bony resorption.

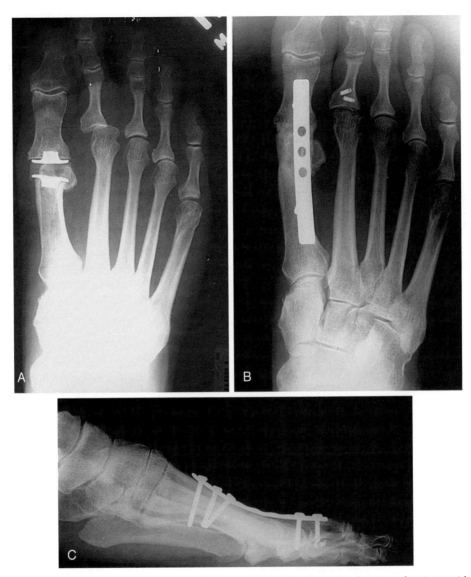

FIGURE 13–11 The shearing of a Silastic implant at the bone/implant interface is considered the principal cause of implant fragmentation and related osteolysis. Metal grommets covering the bone interface, coupled with Silastic implants, were designed to reduce these complications. Early results seem promising. **A:** An anteroposterior radiograph illustrates the use of a metal grommet–docked Silastic implant for arthritis of the first MTP. The first metatarsal has been excessively shortened and, as a result, the patient has developed secondary overload and subluxation of the second MTP joint. **B** and **C:** Because of the severe pain under the second MTP joint, the patient underwent a revision operation involving arthrodesis of the first MTP joint with an intercalary iliac crest bone graft utilizing a plate and screw construct. The second MTP joint dislocation was treated by partial resection of the distal aspect of the proximal phalanx, reduction of the MTP joint, partial excision of the distal metatarsal head, and ligament tightening using two small bone suture anchors in the proximal phalanx.

REFERENCES

1. Lachiewicz PE. Total ankle arthroplasty. Orthop Rev 1994;23:315–320.
2. Stauffer RN, Segal NM. Total ankle arthroplasty: four years' experience. Clin Orthop 1981;160:217–221.
3. Evanski PM, Waugh TR. Management of arthritis of the ankle: an alternative to arthrodesis. Clin Orthop 1977;122:110–115.
4. Weissman BNW, Simmons BP, Thomas WH. Replacement of "other" joints. Radiol Clin North Am 1995;33:355–373.
5. Berquist TH, Kitaoka HB. Foot and ankle. In Berquist TH, ed. Imaging of Orthopedic Appliances and Prostheses. New York: Raven Press, 1995, pp. 575–660.
6. Verhelst MP, Mulier JC, Hoogmartens MJ, et al. Arthrodesis of the ankle joint with complete removal of the distal part of the fibula: experience with the transfibular approach and three different types of fixation. Clin Orthop 1976;118:93–98.
7. Weissman BNW, Sledge CB. Orthopedic Radiology. Philadelphia: WB Saunders, 1986, pp. 589–670.
8. Kile TA, Donnelly RE, Gehrke JC, et al. Tibiotalocalcaneal arthrodesis with an intramedullary device. Foot Ankle Int 1994;15:669–673.
9. Flock TJ, Ishikawa S, Hecht PJ, et al. Heel anatomy for retrograde tibiotalocalcaneal roddings: a roentgenographic and anatomic analysis. Foot Ankle Int 1997;18:233–235.
10. Harper MC, Tisdel CL. Talonavicular arthrodesis for the painful adult-acquired flatfoot. Foot Ankle Int 1996;17:658–661.
11. Graves SC, Mann RA, Graves KO. Triple arthrodesis in older adults. J Bone Joint Surg 1993;75A:355–362.
12. Saltzman CL, El-Khoury GY. The hindfoot alignment view. Foot Ankle Int 1995;16:572–576.
13. Sgarlato TE, Tafuri SA. Digital implant arthroplasty. Clin Podiatr Med Surg 1996;13:255–262.
14. Rosenblum BI, Giurini JM, Chrzan JS, et al. Preventing loss of the great toe with the hallux interphalangeal joint arthroplasty. J Foot Ankle Surg 1994;33:557–560.

14

—

Spinal
Instrumentation

ETHAN J. SCHOCK
GREGORY P. GRAZIANO

Many different implants and techniques have been described for the management of spinal deformity and instability. All share the basic purposes of maintaining a reduction or alignment until bony arthrodesis is achieved. Advances in the understanding of spine biomechanics have allowed for improved design and application of implants. Some of the most common and widely accepted implants are reviewed here.

Posterior Spinal Instrumentation

The evolution of implants used in the treatment of thoracolumbar fractures and deformities has been dictated by the increased appreciation of the importance of maintaining multidirectional stability and restoring normal spinal contours and of the need for strong, low-profile implants.

HARRINGTON INSTRUMENTATION

Harrington instrumentation (Fig. 14–1) has been widely used in the management of thoracolumbar fractures as well as in the correction of other spine deformities. Originally straight, these rods can now be contoured to better approximate the normal curvature of the spine. Rod diameters of 1/8 and 3/16 inch are standard. Built-in ratchet points allow for distraction or compression of the spine. The rods are coupled with the spine by hooks around the base of the transverse processes in the thoracic spine and around the lamina in the lumbar spine.

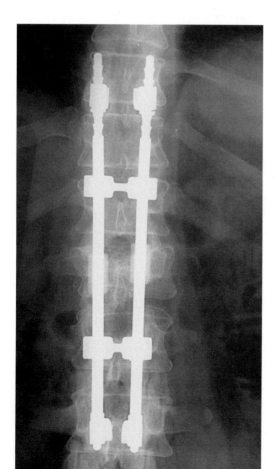

FIGURE 14–1   Harrington distraction instrumentation.

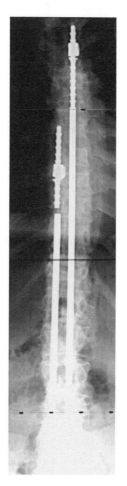

FIGURE 14–2 A failed Harrington rod.

Implant failure is most commonly seen as hook pullout, with an incidence of up to 10%. Additionally, the narrowing of the rod at the first ratchet provides a weak link and concentration of stresses and is the typical point of rod failure (Fig. 14–2).

EDWARDS MODIFICATION OF HARRINGTON IMPLANTS

Edwards and Levine introduced modifications to the Harrington system. Their contourable distraction rods utilize a polyethylene sleeve and L-shaped anatomic laminar hooks that provide simultaneous hyperextension and distraction forces, which eliminate kyphotic deformity. Additionally, this system requires fewer instrumented spinal segments.

JACOBS LOCKING HOOK INSTRUMENTATION

Jacobs and colleagues, in conjunction with the AO group, developed additional modifications to the Harrington instrumentation. The larger (7 mm) contourable rod has threaded ends instead of notches. This allows distraction of the spine but eliminates the decreased strength caused by a notch. Further increase in hook contact area is achieved by the 5-degree tilt of the cranial hook.

This system has been shown to have greater strength than Harrington instrumentation. Possible disadvantages include the need to span at least five motion segments, and this system may not provide adequate fixation for comminuted burst fractures. This system is not recommended for use in the lower spine.

LUQUE SUBLAMINAR WIRES

The popularization of sublaminar wires, L-shaped rods in the management of spinal deformities, is credited to Eduardo Luque (Fig. 14–3). Contoured, 3/16- or 1/4-inch stainless steel or nickel-chrome alloy rods are secured to the spine with 18-gauge sublaminar wires (Fig. 14–4). A variation of this technique employs braided cables that are similarly positioned but have the advantages of increased strength and decreased migration as compared to monofilament wires. This construct has been shown to be superior to Harrington instrumentation in resisting frontal, sagittal, and transverse motion. Additional stability is achieved when the caudal tips are secured to the pelvis (the Galveston technique). The primary mechanical shortcoming of Luque rods and sublaminar wires is compression.

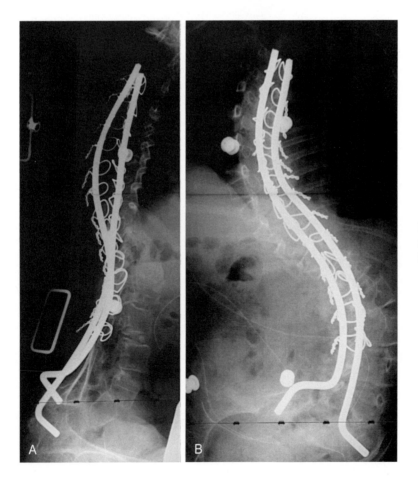

FIGURE 14–3 A and **B:** Luque instrumentation with a Galveston (pelvic) extension.

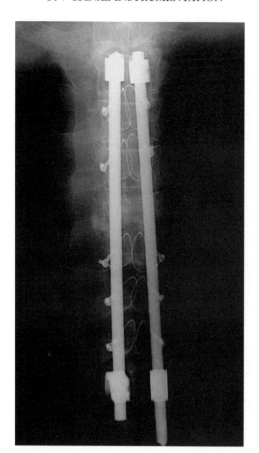

FIGURE 14–4 A TSRH-Luque hybrid construct.

The stability of sublaminar fixation is often combined with other systems, such as Texas Scottish Rite Hospital (TSRH) or Cotrel Dubousset (CD), to create a hybrid construct (see Fig. 14–4). The risk of neurovascular injury during wire placement as well as with wire failure and potential migration has limited the use of this technique to patients with neuromuscular spine deformities.

Failure of this technique is usually noted as fracture or dislocation of the spine immediately above or below the instrumented levels. Continued motion at the operative site can lead to failure of fusion and to pseudarthrosis (Fig. 14–5).

WISCONSIN (DRUMMOND) INTERSPINOUS INSTRUMENTATION

An alternative to sublaminar wire passage was introduced by Drummond, Keene, and Breed (Fig. 14–6). Beaded wires are passed through the base of the spinous processes and through buttons on the opposite sides. This allows for firm fixation of Luque rods and avoids the risk of neurovascular injury that is possible with the passing of sublaminar wires.

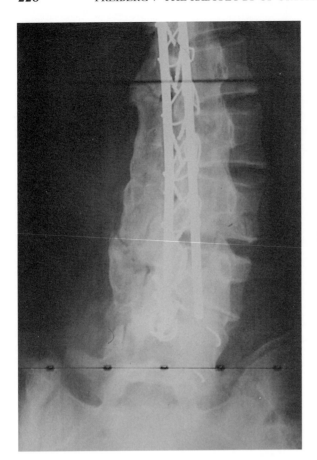

FIGURE 14–5   Luque implants and pseudarthrosis.

FIGURE 14–6   A Harrington-Luque hybrid with Wisconsin wires.

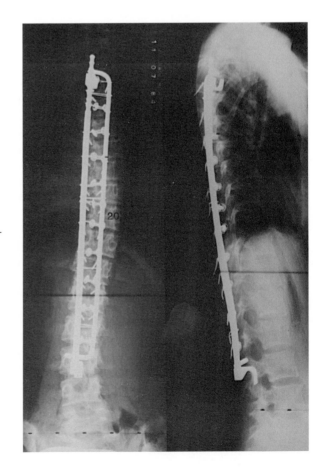

PEDICLE SCREW FIXATION

Roy-Camille and others have employed pedicle screws and plates in the management of thoracolumbar fractures since 1961. More modern systems couple these screws with contoured rods (Fig. 14–7). Standard screws have a 5-mm diameter and are typically 35 mm long. Despite the growing popularity of pedicular fixation in North America and the clinical results that show high fusion rates and low implant failure rates, pedicle screws are classified by the U.S. Food and Drug Administration as class III implants except when used as fusion adjuncts in grade III and IV spondylolisthesis (Fig. 14–8).

With the advent of computerized tomographic (CT; stealth) mapping, placement of cervical pedicle screws became possible. This procedure is technically demanding and is performed only where this new technology is available.

Placement of pedicle screws is challenging and requires intraoperative and postoperative confirmation of screw position. In addition to loss of fixation, disruption of the pedicular cortex can allow canal or foramen compromise with cord or nerve root injury (Figs. 14–9 and 14–10). Encroachment of the screw into adjacent disc spaces can lead to accelerated degeneration of junctional segments. In the lumbar spine, violation of the anterior vertebral cortex jeopardizes the iliac artery and veins.

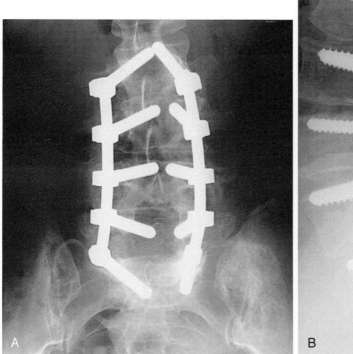
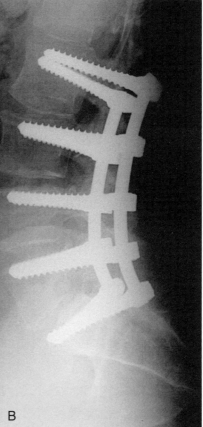

FIGURE 14–7   A and **B:** Pedicle screws in lumbosacral fusion.

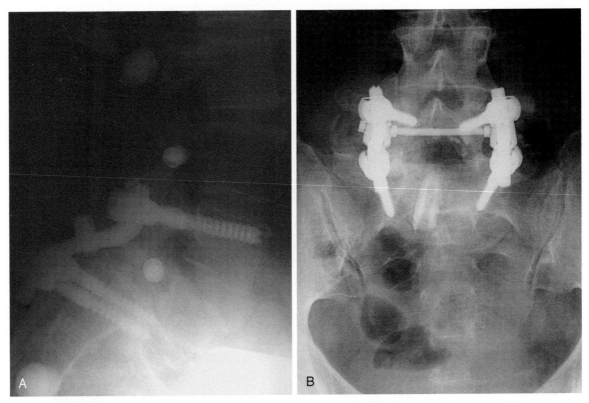

FIGURE 14–8   A and **B:** Contoured rods and pedicle screws for fusion of grade V spondylo-listhesis with visible bone strut graft.

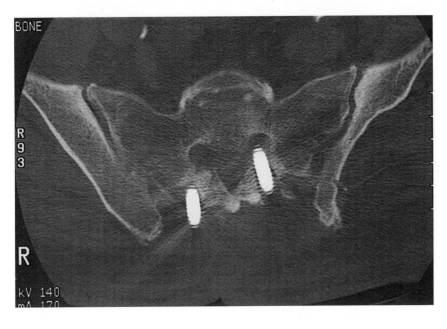

FIGURE 14–9 Axial CT of a pedicle screw in the sacral foramen.

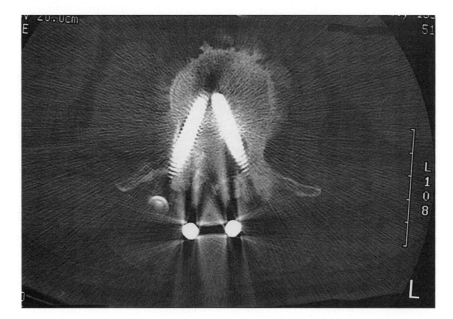

FIGURE 14–10 Axial CT of a pedicle screw in the lumbar foramen.

Pedicle screw failure is seen primarily as breakage of the implant. The failure of the spinal arthrodesis can allow prolonged motion and stress on the implant, causing eventual fatigue and loss of structural integrity (Fig. 14–11).

COMBINED FIXATION DEVICES

Modern instrumentation systems utilize laminar hooks and pedicle screws and can accommodate sublaminar wires. This flexibility offers extremely stable constructs for a variety of indications. These systems (Cotrel-Dubousset, Texas Scottish Rite Hospital, ISOLA) were originally developed for the correction and stabilization of scoliotic curves but are finding increased use for stabilization of thoracolumbar spine fractures. The addition of crossbars between the two rods provides significantly improved stability.

Like other implants, these systems can fail. Radiographic signs of implant failure include broken screws or rods and hook pullout (Figs. 14–12, 14–13, and 14–14). Many systems now offer low-profile hooks and materials that are compatible with magnetic resonance imaging (MRI).

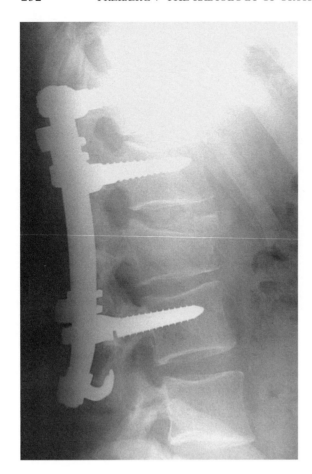

FIGURE 14–11   A broken pedicle screw.

FIGURE 14–12   Pulled-out hook CD instrumentation.

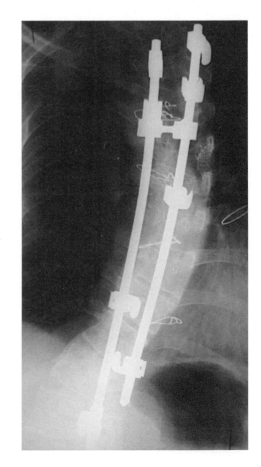

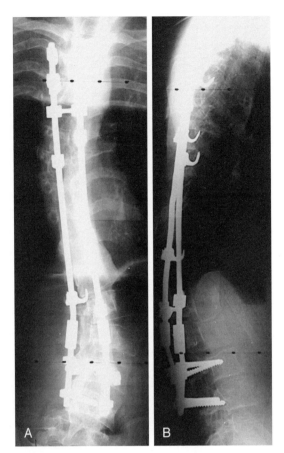

FIGURE 14–13 A and **B:** Pedicle screw pullout and loss of hook fixation in CD instrumentation.

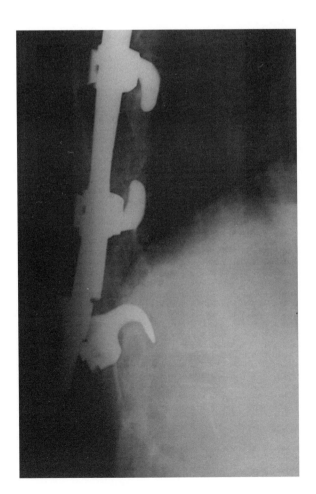

FIGURE 14–14   Dissociation of hook from CD rod.

Anterior Instrumentation

KANEDA INSTRUMENTATION

Kaneda and Gaines introduced a system of implants designed for placement on the lateral aspect of the vertebral body, through an anterior approach (Fig. 14–15). The system employs tetra-spiked plates and 6.25-mm screws to secure smooth rods to the spine. Kaneda instrumentation is often used with an anterior strut graft. Limitations of the system include the increased morbidity likely in an anterior operation, limits in deformity correction, and potential vascular injuries caused by a large anterior device.

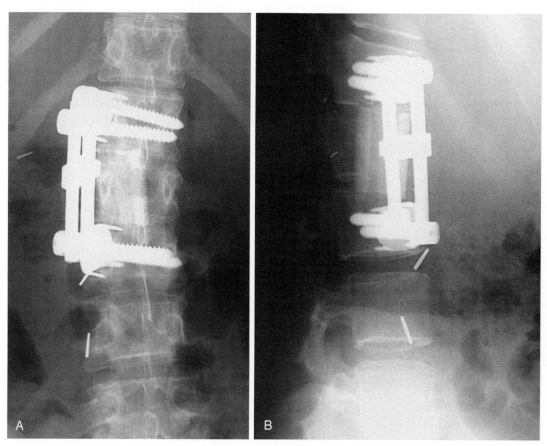

FIGURE 14–15   A and **B:** Kaneda instrumentation.

Z PLATE-ATL FIXATION SYSTEM

This system was developed for the management of thoracolumbar burst fractures and tumors (Fig. 14–16). Its MRI- and CT-compatible titanium plate, bolt, and screw system provides the ability to distract for reduction and to compress bone graft, and it permits anterior loading. Like the Kaneda implant, it is placed on the lateral aspect of the vertebral body. The low profile (3/16 inch) of the device minimizes the risk for vascular injury.

INTERBODY FUSION DEVICES (CAGES)

Lumbar and lumbosacral fusions are increasingly performed with cage-type devices. These implants are positioned at the desired disc level through an anterior approach. The hollow device has holes allowing the contained bone graft to contribute to the interbody fusion mass. Variations of design include cylindrical (BAK) (Fig. 14–17) and tapered (TIF) implants as well as threaded cortical bone allografts, which function in the same manner.

Many other systems of anterior spinal fixation exist as well, including the Zielke, Syracuse I Plate, and TSRH systems.

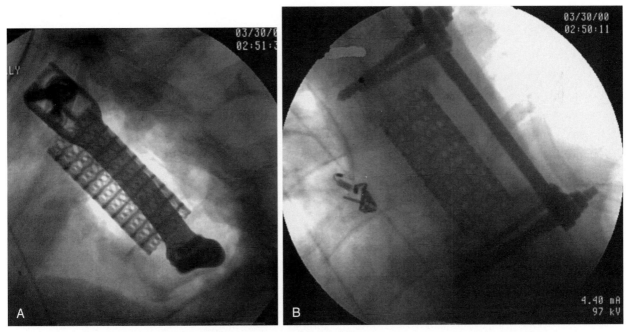

FIGURE 14–16 A and **B:** Z plate-ATL fixation system and paramesh anterior strut in thoracic corpectomy and fusion. (Courtesy Danek, Memphis, TN)

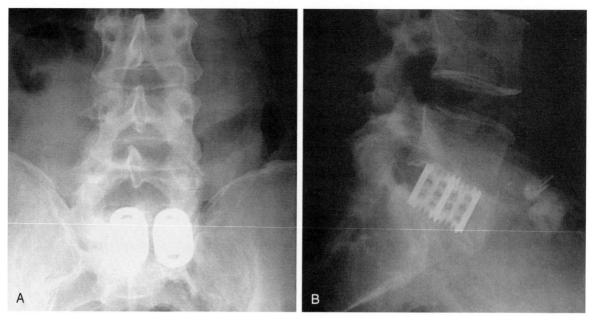

FIGURE 14–17   A and **B:** Interbody cages (BAK).

Cervical Instrumentation and Implants

The complex anatomy of the cervical spine and its many different fracture patterns require multiple techniques and devices for stabilization. The complexity ranges from basic wiring and bone grafting of adjacent segments to precisely placed, fluoroscopically guided transarticular screws. However, the goals of restoration of normal alignment and structural stability that allow for solid fusion and permanent protection of neural structures remain constant.

POSTERIOR INTERSPINOUS WIRING

Multiple wiring techniques have been described. Most utilize the lamina (in the upper cervical segments), the spinous processes, or both, to anchor the wires. The incorporation of posterior, intersegmental bone blocks provides additional stability, especially to extension.

In the Gallie technique, 20-gauge wire is utilized to secure corticocancellous bone graft to the lamina of C1 and the spinous process of C2.

Similar to the Gallie procedure, the Brooks and Jenkins technique uses two wires to secure the lamina of C1 to C2 (Fig. 14–18). Additionally, corticocancellous bone block graft is placed between the laminae, providing additional stability. This method decreases the posteriorly directed vector force and is useful for maintaining reduction of unstable type II odontoid fractures.

In the Bohlman triple-wire technique, a midline 20-gauge wire is secured through drill holes in the spinous processes of adjacent cervical segments. Two 22-gauge wires are then utilized to hold two unicortical bone grafts to the posterior elements of the involved vertebrae. This technique is commonly used in lower cervical spine arthrodeses.

In oblique facet wiring (Fig. 14–19), unilateral or bilateral wiring of the articular masses of a "jumped" vertebra to the spinous process of the intact caudal vertebra provides stability in the presence of rotational and flexion forces.

The Halifax clamp is a variation of the posterior wiring technique (Fig. 14–20). This device combines lightweight metal hooks with the compression potential of interspinous wiring.

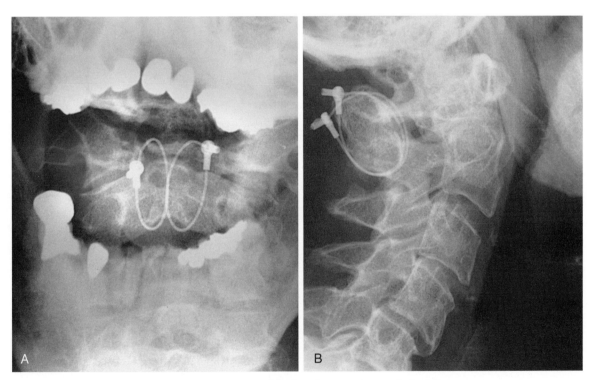

FIGURE 14–18   A and B: Brooks posterior cervical wiring.

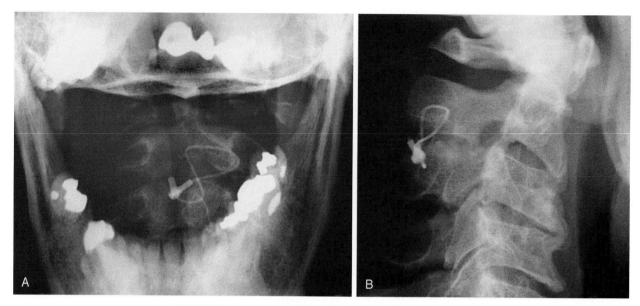

FIGURE 14–19 **A** and **B:** Oblique cervical facet wiring.

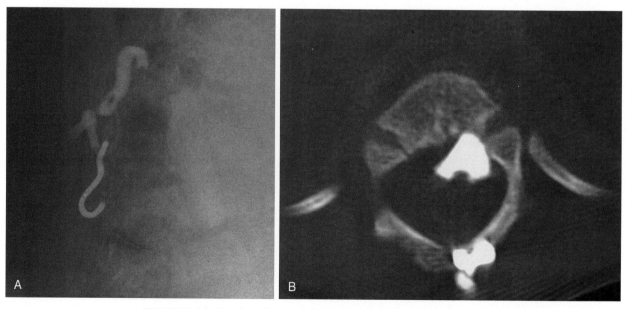

FIGURE 14–20 **A** and **B:** Halifax clamp and displaced strut graft.

C1–C2 TRANSARTICULAR SCREW FIXATION
(MAGERL SCREWS)

Atlantoaxial instability and unstable odontoid fractures are indications for Magerl screws (Fig. 14–21). Cephalad-directed 3.5-mm cannulated screws are introduced from the laminar isthmus of C2 into the lateral masses of C1. This exacting procedure requires fluoroscopic guidance.

POSTERIOR CERVICAL PLATING

Plates and screws are frequently used to provide rigid internal fixation of the cervical spine (Fig. 14–22). Lateral mass screws secure the plates to the spine, allowing for stabilization in the presence of severe instability or when deficient posterior elements preclude interspinous wiring. Small plates allow for rigid fixation of single motion segments, or multiple segments (including the occiput) can be secured (Fig. 14–23). Screw backout and loosening are the primary signs of implant and procedure failure. The addition of posterior instrumentation is occasionally made in cases of failed or inadequate anterior procedures (Fig. 14–24).

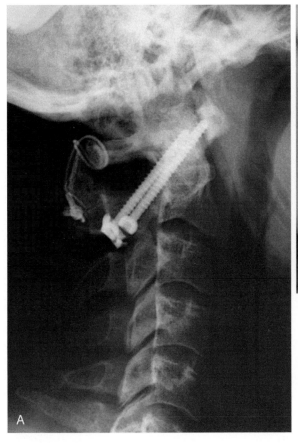

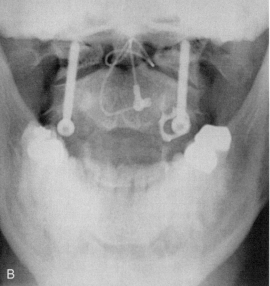

FIGURE 14–21 **A** and **B:** C1–C2 transarticular (Magerl) screws.

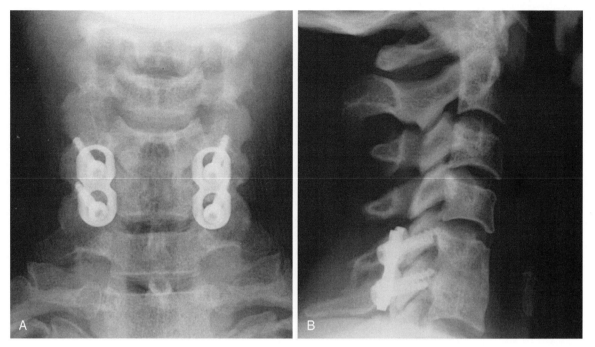

FIGURE 14–22   **A** and **B:** Posterior cervical plates.

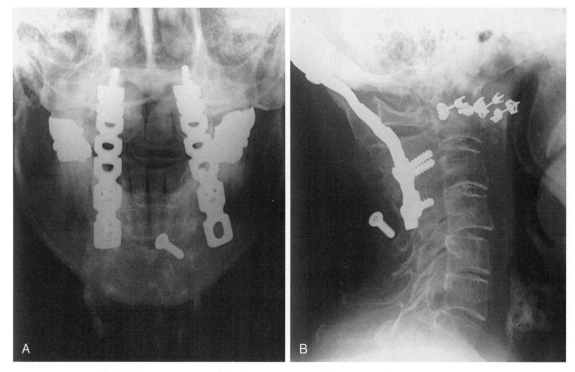

FIGURE 14–23   **A** and **B:** Occipito-cervical fusion in a rheumatoid patient.

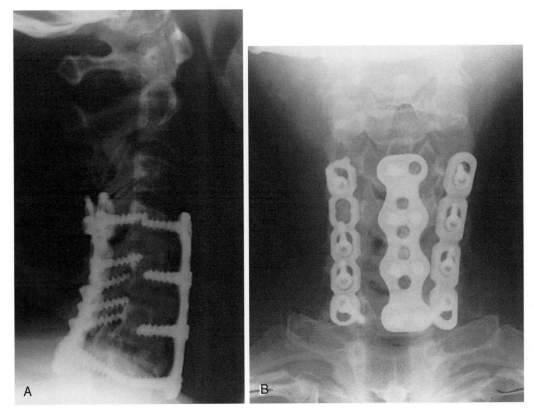

FIGURE 14–24   **A** and **B:** Combined anterior and posterior cervical plating.

ANTERIOR SCREW FIXATION OF THE DENS (ETTER)

In the setting of a transverse, unstable dens fracture with a stable atlas, one or two cannulated 3.5-mm screws may be utilized to maintain reduction. Failure of bone healing and other complications are not uncommon in this procedure. They are most commonly encountered with improper screw positioning or with inadequate bone stock as seen when treating dens fracture nonunions.

ANTERIOR CERVICAL DISCECTOMY AND FUSION

Arthrodesis of the cervical spine through an anterior approach is commonly achieved with anterior cervical discectomy and fusion (ACDF) through placement of a cortico-cancellous allograft or autograft (Fig. 14–25). The use of an anterior plate has the additional benefits of greater stability and decreased extrusion of the graft. Proximity to vital neck structures demands that these plates have a low profile and be securely fixated. The Atlantis plate system (Danek, Memphis, TN) has locking, countersunk screws and is made of titanium, allowing future MRI (Fig. 14–26).

Radiographic signs of failure include extrusion or collapse of bone graft and loosening or backout of screws.

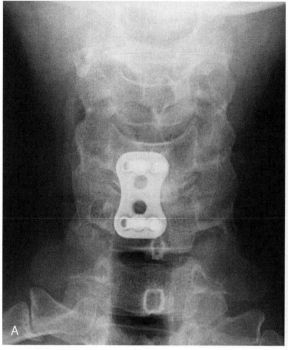

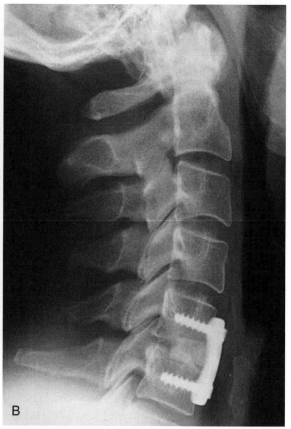

FIGURE 14–25   A and **B:** C5–C6 ACDF with graft.

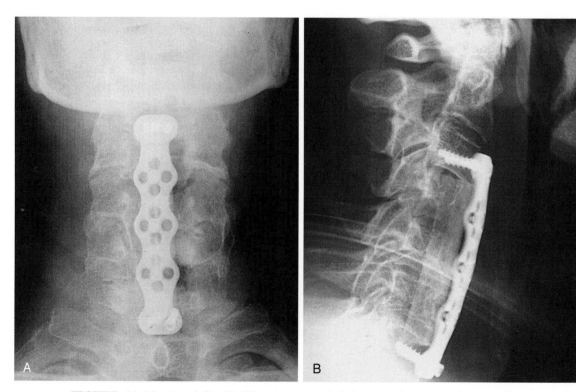

FIGURE 14–26   A and **B:** C3–C7 anterior cervical fusion with strut graft and inferior screw backout.

BIBLIOGRAPHY

Amstutz HC, Ouzounian T, Grauer D, et al. The grid radiograph: a simple technique for consistent high-resolution visualization of the hip. J Bone Joint Surg 1986;68A:1052–1056.

Baldursson H, Egund N, Hansson LI, et al. Instability and wear of total hip prostheses determined with roentgen stereophotogrammetry. Arch Orthop Trauma Surg 1979;95:257–263.

Baldursson H, Hansson LI, Olsson TH, et al. Migration of the acetabular socket after total hip replacement determined by roentgen stereophotogrammetry. Acta Orthop Scand 1980;51:535–540.

Charnley J, Cupic Z. The nine- and ten-year results of the low-friction arthroplasty of the hip. Clin Orthop 1973;95:9–25.

Charnley J, Halley DK. Rate of wear in total hip replacement. Clin Orthop 1975;112:170–179.

Charnley J, Kamangar A, Longfield MD. The optimum size of prosthetic heads in relation to the wear of plastic sockets in total replacement of the hip. Med Biol Eng 1969;7:31–39.

Clarac JP, Pries P, Launay L, et al. Erosion of polyethylene cupulae: radiological study of 123 Charnley total prostheses. Rev Chir Orthop 1986;72:97–100.

Clarke IC, Black K, Rennie C, et al. Can wear in total hip arthroplasties be assessed from radiographs? Clin Orthop 1976;121:126–142.

Clarke IC, Gruen TA, Matos M, et al. Improved methods for quantitative radiographic evaluation with particular reference to total-hip arthroplasty. Clin Orthop 1976;121:83–91.

Devane PA. The measurement of polyethylene wear in metal-backed acetabular components. Master of Science thesis, University of Western Ontario London, Ontario, Canada, 1993.

Devane PA, Bourne RB, Rorabeck CH, et al. Measurement of polyethylene wear in metal-backed acetabular cups. I. Three-dimensional technique. Clin Orthop 1995;319:303–316.

Franzen H, Mjoberg B. Wear and loosening of the hip prosthesis: a roentgen stereophotogrammetric 3-year study of 14 cases. Acta Orthop Scand 1990;6:499–501.

Griffith MJ, Seidenstein MK, Williams D, et al. Socket wear in Charnley low-friction arthroplasty of the hip. Clin Orthop 1978;137:37–47.

Herrlin K, Selvik G, Pettersson H. Space orientation of total hip prosthesis: a method for three-dimensional determination. Acta Radiol Diagn Stockh 1986;27:619–627.

Ilchmann T. Radiographic assessment of cup migration and wear after hip replacement. Acta Orthop Scand Suppl 1997;276:1–26.

Jones PR, Taylor CJ, Hukins DW, et al. Prosthetic hip failure: preliminary findings of retrospective radiograph image analysis. Eng Med 1988;17:119–125.

Jones PR, Taylor CJ, Hukins DW, et al. Prosthetic hip failure: retrospective radiograph image analysis of the acetabular cup. J Biomed Eng 1989;11:253–257.

Livermore J, Ilstrup D, Morrey B. Effect of femoral head size on wear of the polyethylene acetabular component. J Bone Joint Surg 1990;72A:518–528.

Martell JM, Berdia S. Determination of polyethylene wear in total hip replacements with use of digital radiographs. J Bone Joint Surg 1997;79A:1635–1641.

Selvik G. A roentgen stereophotogrammetric method for study of the kinematics of the skeletal system. Doctor of Philosophy thesis, University of Lund, Sweden, 1974.

Selvik G, Alberius P, Aronson AS. A roentgen stereophotogrammetric system: construction, calibration and technical accuracy. Acta Radiol Diagn Stockh 1983;24:343–352.

Shaver SM, Brown TD, Hillis SL, et al. Digital edge-detection measurement of polyethylene wear after total hip arthroplasty. J Bone Joint Surg 1997;79A:690–700.

Walker PS, Salvati EA. The measurement and effects of friction and wear in artificial hip joints. J Biomed Mater Res 1973;7:327–342.

Wientroub S, Boyde A, Chrispin AR, et al. The use of stereophotogrammetry to measure acetabular and femoral anteversion. J Bone Joint Surg 1981;63B:209–213.

Wroblewski BM. Direction and rate of socket wear in Charnley low-friction arthroplasty. J Bone Joint Surg 1985;67B:757–761.

Index

Note: Page numbers in *italics* refer to illustrations; page numbers followed by (t) refer to tables.

E

Edwards modification, of Harrington
  instrumentation, 225
Elbow, fracture of, wire fixation of, *43*
Elbow replacement surgery, 22
  bone loss/osteolysis following, *24*
  constrained implant in, 22, *24*
  nonconstrained implant in, 22, *22*
  semiconstrained implant in, 22, *23*
Electrical stimulator, in treatment of
    nonunion of fracture, in femur, *54*
  in hand or wrist, *35*
Endobutton, stabilization of hamstring
    graft with, in reconstruction of
    anterior cruciate ligament of knee,
    63, 65
External fixation, of fractures, 39, *39–41.*
    See also *Rod(s), external.*

F

Fabellofibular ligament, 60
Feet. See *Foot.*
Femoral augment(s), in revision
    arthroplasty of knee, *170*
Femoral component(s), in hip replacement
    surgery. See also *Femoral head
    component; Femoral stem component.*
  evaluation of, 96, *96*
  hydroxyapatite-coated, 153–156, *153–
    156*
    radiolucent lines around, 153, *153,
      155*
  loosening of, 98, *104, 105, 125*
  neutral position of, 96, *96, 100*
  osteolysis at site of, *108, 117, 120,
    122, 126, 129*
  radiolucent lines around, 97, *97*
  revision of, 131
    diaphyseal press-fit–dependent de-
      vice in, 131, *131*
    impaction allografting with cement
      in, 131–134, *132, 134, 135*
    complications of, 133, *133*
Femoral head component, in hip
    replacement surgery. See also
    Femoral stem component.
  acetabular malposition uncovering,
    115
  dislocation of, *114*
  protrusion of, into acetabular prosthe-
    sis, *109, 124*
  socket for. See *Hip replacement surgery,
    acetabular component in.*
Femoral stem component, in hip
    replacement surgery. See also
    Femoral head component.
  cement fractures surrounding, *5*
  fracture of, *112*
  modes of failure of, 97
  radiography of, 3, *4*
    demonstrating cement fractures, *5*
    displaying implant fracture, *112*
  substitution of new implant for, 131
    diaphyseal press-fit–dependent de-
      vice in, 131, *131*
    impaction allografting with cement
      in, 131–134, *132, 134, 135*

Femoral stem component *(Continued)*
    complications of, 133, *133*
Femoral tunnel, in reconstruction of
    anterior cruciate ligament of knee,
    59, *63, 64, 65*
  problems with positioning of, *67*
Femur, comminuted fracture of, screw and
    sideplate fixation of, *45, 47*
  fracture of, 39
    comminuted, screw and sideplate fixa-
      tion of, *45, 47*
    electrical stimulation of union of, *54*
    intramedullary nailing of, 54, *56*
    plate fixation of. See *Femur, screw fixa-
      tion of.*
    screw fixation of, at level of hip, *44,
      45, 46*
      intramedullary nailing and, *56*
      problems with, *45, 113*
      at supracondylar level, with side-
        plate attachment, *47*
  head of, prosthetic. See *Femoral head
    component, in hip replacement surgery.*
  neck of, fracture of, 39
    screw fixation of, *46*
      intramedullary nailing and, *56*
      problems with, *113*
    supracondylar fracture of, screw fixation
      of, with sideplate attachment, *47*
Fibula, fracture of, plate fixation of, *48*
  screw fixation of, *48*
Fingers. See also *Hand.*
  replacement of joints of, with silicone
    implant, *30*
  tendon attachment in, suture anchor mi-
    gration following, *36*
First metatarsal–cuneiform arthrodesis,
    218
First metatarsal osteotomy, for hallux
    valgus, *218*
First metatarsophalangeal joint, fusion of,
    failed silicone implant as indication
    for, *221*
  hallus valgus as indication for, *219*
  plate-and-screw fixation of, failed sili-
    cone implant as indication for, *221*
  replacement of, with metal/polyethylene
    implant, for arthritis, *220*
    with silicone implant, for arthritis,
      220, 221
      problems with, *220, 221*
Fixation, of fractures. See specific repairs,
    e.g., *Screw fixation.*
Fluid, at or near prosthetic hip,
    ultrasonographic features of, *193, 194*
Foot. See also *Ankle.*
  deformities of, 217
    treatment of, 217, *217–219*
  toes of, deformities of, 219
    implants for, 219
    improper angulation between, 217
      treatment of, 217, *218, 219*
Forefoot, deformities of, 217
  treatment of, 217, *218, 219*
Fracture(s), 39
  acetabular, *5*
    plate fixation of, *50, 51*
  ankle, plate fixation of, *48*

Fracture(s) *(Continued)*
    screw fixation of, *48, 49*
      revascularization following, Haw-
        kins' sign as evidence of, *49*
    axial, involving odontoid process, screw
      fixation of, 241
  cement, following hip replacement sur-
    gery, *5, 104, 116, 123*
  comminuted, of femur, screw and side-
    plate fixation of, *45, 47*
    of humerus, plate fixation of, *82*
    of tibial plateau, screw-plate-and-wire
      fixation of, *53*
  C2 vertebral, involving odontoid pro-
    cess, screw fixation of, 241
  dens axis, screw fixation of, 241
  diaphyseal, of humerus, plate fixation of,
    84
    of radius, plate fixation of, *32*
      screw fixation of, *32*
    of tibia, pin and rod fixation of, *39*
    of ulna, plate fixation of, *32*
      screw fixation of, *32*
  distal radial, pin and rod fixation of, *33*
    plate fixation of, *34*
    screw fixation of, *34*
    wire fixation of, *42*
  distal tibial, intramedullary nailing of,
    56
    ring fixation of, *41*
  elbow, wire fixation of, *43*
  external fixation of, 39, *39–41.* See also
    Rod(s), external.
  femoral, 39
    comminuted, screw and sideplate fixa-
      tion of, *45, 47*
    electrical stimulation of union of, *54*
    intramedullary nailing of, 54, *56*
    plate fixation of. See *Fracture(s), femo-
      ral, screw fixation of.*
    screw fixation of, at level of hip, *44,
      45, 46*
      intramedullary nailing and, *56*
      problems with, *45, 113*
      at supracondylar level, with side-
        plate attachment, *47*
  femoral stem, following hip replace-
    ment, *112*
  fibular, plate fixation of, *48*
    screw fixation of, *48*
  fixation of. See specific repairs, e.g.,
    Screw fixation.
  hand, nonunion of, electrical stimula-
    tion in treatment of, *35*
    plate fixation of, *36*
    screw fixation of, *36*
    wire fixation of, *35*
  heterotopic ossification following, *200*
    scintigraphic evidence for, *201*
  hip, screw fixation of. See under *Frac-
    ture(s), femoral.*
  hip socket. See *Fracture(s), acetabular.*
  humeral, arthroplasty for, *83*
    blade plate fixation of, *82*
    comminuted, plate fixation of, *82*
    diaphyseal, plate fixation of, *84*
    intramedullary nailing of, *81*
    pin fixation of, *80*